LOVE, MEDICINE & MIRACLES

Lessons Learned About Self-Healing
from a Surgeon's Experience
with Exceptional Patients

Bernie S. Siegel, M.D.

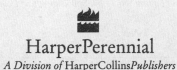

HarperPerennial
A Division of HarperCollinsPublishers

Copyright acknowledgments appear on pages 240–241.

A hardcover edition of this book was published in 1986 by Harper & Row, Publishers, Inc.

HarperCollins books may be purchased for educational, business, or sales promotional use. For information please write: Special Markets Department, Harper-Collins Publishers, Inc., 10 East 53rd Street, New York, NY 10022.

First HarperPerennial edition published 1990.
Reissued 1998.

Designed by C. Linda Dingler

Library of Congress Cataloging-in-Publication Data

Siegel, Bernie S.
    Love, medicine & miracles : lessons learned about self-healing from a
surgeon's experience with exceptional patients / Bernie S. Siegel.
        p. cm. ill.
    Includes bibliographical references.
    ISBN 0–06–091983-3
    1. Medicine and psychology. 2. Love. 3. Mind and body. 4. Attitude to
Health—popular works. 5. Neoplasms—psychology—popular works.
6. Psychophysiology—popular works. 7. Self Care—psychology—popular works.
I. Title.
R726.5.S54 1990
615.5—dc20   89–46437

98 99 00 01 02 RRD   50 49 48 47 46 45 44 43 42

To the Act of Creation

To my parents, Si and Rose, for showing me how to love and hope

To my wife, Bobbie, for putting up with me and for always being there to learn from and love

To her parents, Merle and Ado, for their courage and humor

To our children, Jonathan, Jeffrey, Stephen, and the twins, Carolyn and Keith, for all the love and beauty they have brought into our lives

To all my exceptional associates, patients, and friends for taking the time to teach, support, and accept me

To Victoria Pryor, Carol Cohen, Gary Selden— acknowledging how much love, acceptance, and forgiveness a surgeon requires to complete a book

Contents

Illustrations follow page 116.

Reflections and Thoughts on
Love, Medicine & Miracles

There are several things I am happy to share with you since the writing of *Love, Medicine & Miracles.*

I retired from the practice of surgery in 1989, because by that time more health care professionals were willing to listen to my message. Once they understood that my work had a scientific basis, they were willing to accept it. I no longer had to keep explaining myself but could instead share my experience and therefore help more people by what I had learned. Ten or twenty years ago if they listened, they were more likely to argue about the validity of what I was saying. I appeared on all the talk shows as an excellent source of conflict and controversy. There was much misunderstanding of the statements I made regarding the role of illness in a person's life. I spent a good deal of time defending myself and explaining what I meant. The point I was trying to make related to the fact that an illness had effects on a person's life beyond just the physical dimension. There were beneficial side effects and a freedom to live that some people obtained from their disease because it made them aware of their mortality. Since we are all mortal, why did some people need to be ill to have the freedom to live their unique lives and experience the beneficial side effects?

Today the health professionals and talk shows are asking for information. I am more often a source of inspiration, not inflammation. Both doctors and patients need healing and are far more ready to listen and learn today. As a matter of fact, I recently read a very moving book by a physician whose wife died of cancer. In the book he apologizes to me. Now, he and I never met and he has nothing to apologize for, except his previous beliefs. The message he shares through his writing is that he has learned that his family had a unique and difficult experience, not just a diagnosis that one prescribed treatment for. My teachings and meditations were important to him and his wife as they lived the experience. Suddenly hope and love became very important complementary therapies.

Before writing this introduction I reread my previously published books and was not disappointed by what I read. There is a good deal of important and useful information within them. They are good training manuals for those facing adversity. I am even wiser today, due to my further experience with adversity and what I have learned since writing these books and starting Exceptional Cancer Patients in 1978. I want to share what I have learned in the intervening time.

One of the things I have learned is that I haven't discovered anything new about survival behavior. The message is an age-old one and can be found in the words of the prophets of the past and those struggling to survive today's difficulties, from exceptional patients to members of Alcoholics Anonymous and the Marines. Science and medicine certainly have confirmed through recent research the personality profile and psychology associated with survival behavior and how they affect the body's chemistry and healing ability.

Information about healing and surviving has been handed down to us for thousands of years by all the great prophets and spiritual leaders. What I have learned is that their message is similar to my own. When one finds a common theme in the writings of those who are healers, one knows there is truth in them. If I were rewriting my books today I would be sure to include the messages of these healers and the most recent scientific support of the advantages of this kind of behavior and lifestyle.

If I were rewriting *Love, Medicine & Miracles*, I might consider changing its title to *The Side Effects of Cancer*. Healing is hard work, as is any change one must make in one's life. I and others have learned, however, that the side effects of cancer may not all be bad ones. Yes, cancer can kill and we tend to think of side effects as problems, but there are good side effects too. An awareness of one's mortality can lead you to wake up and live an authentic, meaningful life. I can read you an article entitled "Thank God I Have Cancer." The 'Thank God' is for the time the cancer gave the author to learn about the beauty, kindness and love that are here for us to share. These side effects also produce a longer life as their byproduct.

The ugly duckling had to do a lot of personal work to find himself and his beauty and to heal his life. He had no support from his family or health professionals to help him find self-esteem and love. He found it in his reflection. I feel that a patient should not have to go through the same struggle. One's family and the medical profession should be able to educate and instruct about appropriate survival behavior when adversity, in the form of an illness, occurs in life. The issue is not about living forever and testing God, but utilizing all of the physical and emotional forces available for healing. The mind and body are not separate units, but one integrated system. How we act and what we think, eat, and feel are all related to our health. Physicians should be capable of teaching this behavior to patients. I spend more time teaching now than ever, and my most grateful patients are the ones who thank me for teaching them how to deal with all of life's difficulties, not just the physical ones.

Medical education does not deal with many of the difficulties physicians must confront in themselves and their patients. Physicians need to be good technicians and know how to prescribe, but for healing to occur they also need to incorporate philosophy and spirituality into their treatment. We need to feel as well as think. When one's existence is threatened there are more issues and questions to confront than what medicine to take, or operation to undergo. As one woman wrote, we need a mutual investment society—the patient and the doctors investing in each other.

So how do you display survival behavior and find a good doctor who knows how to use his or her expertise and be your teacher? Ask the doctor if he or she has ever been criticized by his or her family, patients or nurses. If the answer is yes, that is the doctor to use. Why? Because that is someone there is hope for. You don't criticize someone you don't think is willing to listen, learn and hopefully change. As the poet Rumi said, "Your criticism polishes my mirror." Good doctors understand this. The nurses also know the capable, caring physicians from their experience with them, so ask their opinion and don't hesitate to speak up if you are not treated with respect. Submissive behavior is not survival behavior. Be the human being, not the diagnosis or room number.

I mentioned that as I reviewed my previous writings I felt satisfied with the content. My next feeling was simply remembering the many wonderful and loving people who were and still are my teachers. Now that I am not sitting down with them for several hours each week, I miss them, and rereading their stories really brought that home to me.

So many religions and philosophies tell us how to find our way or path. What they are all trying to tell us is to pay attention to our feelings and let them guide us. If you ignore your body and its messages, at some point you will suffer the consequences. Two of Christ's messages sum it up very well. "He who seeks to save his life will lose it, and he who is willing to lose his life will save it." I interpret this to mean that we lose our authentic life when we give in to the demands of others, or we become something others want us to be in order to gain their love or simply continue to be cared for. When we awaken to our mortality, we refuse to live the life that is killing us and start living and being our true selves. On a practical level it may mean changing occupations, moving, healing or ending relationships and bringing meaning and a new attitude into life and working for the right Lord.

Your life is stored in your body. Christ's second message is, "If you do not bring forth what is within you, what you do not bring forth will destroy you. If you bring forth what is within you, what you bring forth will save you." He is talking about our feelings and body memories, and is quite correct.

The earliest spiritual writings tell us to sit quietly and listen. The Kabbalah gives specific instructions on how to hear the voice of God and be enlightened so that your wisdom can be used to help others. Survivors take time to be still and listen.

You may call it meditation, imagery, relaxation or journal writing but it all amounts to finding time to be still and listen to the voice within you and the voice which will come to you. I often have this experience when I am out jogging or bicycling by myself with nothing to distract me. Take the time to listen. If you listen, you will learn your purpose here and be able to die joyfully, knowing that you have served in your way and fulfilled the reasons for your creation. Survivors deal with the spiritual, existential and emotional aspects of their lives. When we commit ourselves to egoless, unconditional love, true healing begins. We are then not devoted to changing people but devoted to the people. Love itself is a miraculous healing force. In a sense it is the miracle and the reason for being. So ask yourself what lesson you are here to learn and learn that lesson by the way you distribute your love to the world. Remember the blindness of love does great things to obliterate the wounds of the world.

We say love is blind because it helps us to see the world in a way that is significant for survival. Love's blindness is therapeutic because it allows us to function without storing the images of life's difficulties within us. I tell people, "If you can't love at least develop amnesia so you can live a more peaceful life, unable to remember all the things people did to upset you. I am here to help you survive and so is our creator." If God weren't intelligent, loving energy then none of us would be here today. The ability to heal has been built into us and into all living things. God doesn't play favorites. We get upset when bacteria become resistant to antibiotics, but not by our ability to become resistant to disease. They are both survival mechanisms put there by our creator to sustain life in a balanced way.

Do not live a role. Live an authentic life. Many people die when they can't work anymore due to their illness. They do not see relationships as providing another reason for living. On the other hand a mother of nine may not die because of her children but the year after they leave home she dies. Find your life and live it. Do not live a role.

Please remember that information doesn't change anyone. Inspiration does. Find your reason to live. Be inspired by it and undergo revelation and transformation. I have found only one bit of information that could help change you. It is that you are mortal and will die some day. Therefore, don't do things to not die but do things to enhance the quality of your life and you may be surprised by how long you do live. Accept that you will die and make decisions about how you want to spend the limited amount of time you have. Then you won't need to go into therapy in Heaven to deal with the bitterness and resentment over all the things you did and then died anyway.

Learn from the wisdom of others and enjoy your life experience. Remember the Bible ends in Revelations, not Conclusions, and graduations are commencements not terminations. Please let this book be a revelation to you and let me be your guide to transformation and a life of peace, love and healing. Begin now.

Bernie S. Siegel, M.D.

Introduction

Several years ago a group of nurses at a nearby hospital asked
me to talk to Jonathan, a physician who had just been diagnosed as having lung cancer. He had been admitted in good
physical condition and was in good humor, joking with all the
nurses. When he learned his diagnosis, however, he became
terribly depressed and withdrawn.

I talked with him about the relationship between attitude
and disease. I discussed Norman Cousins's experience with
suspected tuberculosis as he described it in *Anatomy of an
Illness:*

My first experience in coping with a bleak medical diagnosis
came at the age of ten, when I was sent to a tuberculosis
sanitarium. I was terribly frail and underweight, and it seemed
logical to suppose that I was in the grip of a serious malady. Later
it was discovered that the doctors had mistakenly interpreted
normal calcification as TB markings. X-rays at that time were not
yet a totally reliable basis for complex diagnosis. In any case, I
spent six months at the sanitarium.

What was most interesting to me about that early experience
was that patients divided themselves into two groups: those who
were confident they would beat back the disease and be able to
resume normal lives, and those who resigned themselves to a
prolonged and even fatal illness. Those of us who held to the
optimistic view became good friends, involved ourselves in
creative activities, and had little to do with the patients who had
resigned themselves to the worst. When newcomers arrived at
the hospital, we did our best to recruit them before the bleak
brigade went to work.

I couldn't help being impressed with the fact that the boys in my group had a far higher percentage of "discharged as cured" outcomes than the kids in the other group. Even at the age of ten, I was being philosophically conditioned; I became aware of the power of the mind in overcoming disease. The lessons I learned about hope at that time played an important part in my complete recovery and in the feelings I have had since about the preciousness of life.

Jonathan told me, "I know about that. I had tuberculosis myself and was told I'd be in the sanatorium for two years. I said, 'No, I'll be home for Christmas with my family.' And in fact, in six months, on December 23, I was discharged."

I assured him, "You can do the same thing with cancer," but in two weeks he was dead. His wife thanked me for my efforts and explained that her husband hadn't wanted to fight for recovery because his life and work had lost all meaning.

Sir William Osler, the brilliant Canadian physician and medical historian, said that the outcome of tuberculosis had more to do with what went on in the patient's mind than what went on in his lungs. He was echoing Hippocrates, who said he would rather know what sort of person has a disease than what sort of disease a person has. Louis Pasteur and Claude Bernard, two of the giants of nineteenth-century biology, argued all their lives whether the most important factor in disease was the "soil"—the human body—or the germ. On his deathbed, Pasteur admitted that Bernard had been right, declaring, "It is the soil."

Despite the insights of these eminent doctors, medicine still focuses on disease, giving it a failure orientation. Its practitioners still act as though disease catches people, rather than understanding that people catch disease by becoming susceptible to the seeds of illness to which we are all constantly exposed. Although the best physicians have always known better, medicine as a whole has rarely studied the people who *don't* get sick. Most doctors seldom consider how a patient's attitude towards life shapes that life's quantity and quality.

Patients vary enormously. Some will do almost anything rather than alter their lives to increase their chances for a cure.

When I offer them a choice between an operation and a change in lifestyle, eight out of ten say, "Operate. It hurts less. That way all I have to do is get a babysitter for the week I'm in the hospital." At the other extreme are those I call exceptional patients, or survivors. They refuse to participate in defeat—like one woman in my care, a blind diabetic amputee with cancer, who has lived longer than statistics would have predicted and now spends much of her time on the phone cheering up *other* patients. She and other exceptional patients have taught me that the mind can dramatically affect the body and that the ability to love is not limited by bodily illness.

Freud's theory that our instinct for self-preservation is opposed by some sort of death instinct has been rejected by many later psychologists. However, we all know that many people live their lives as though trying to cut them short. Exceptional patients have overcome the pressures, conflicts, and habits that lead others to act from this conscious or unconscious "death wish." Instead, their every thought and deed advances the cause of life. I personally feel that we do have biological "live" and "die" mechanisms within us. Other doctors' scientific research and my own day-to-day clinical experience have convinced me that the state of the mind changes the state of the body by working through the central nervous system, the endocrine system, and the immune system. Peace of mind sends the body a "live" message, while depression, fear, and unresolved conflict give it a "die" message. Thus, all healing is scientific, even if science can't yet explain exactly how the unexpected "miracles" occur.

Exceptional patients manifest the will to live in its most potent form. They take charge of their lives even if they were never able to before, and they work hard to achieve health and peace of mind. They do not rely on doctors to take the initiative but rather use them as members of a team, demanding the utmost in technique, resourcefulness, concern, and open-mindedness. If they're not satisfied, they change doctors.

However, exceptional patients also are loving, and thus understand the difficulties a physician faces. In most cases, my advice to a dissatisfied patient is to give the doctor a hug.

Usually this makes the doctor more willing to respond to the patient's needs, because you *become* an individual to your physician and are *treated* as an individual, not a disease. You become what I affectionately term "crazy." One patient told me she went back to her doctor with my advice but couldn't bring herself to hug him. "Instead," she said, "I gave him the most compassionate look I could. And you know what? He sat down, told me he needed to lose weight and get more exercise, and then *he* hugged *me!*" If the hug doesn't work, however, then it's time to get another doctor, because I know patients who are literally being killed by their relationship with their doctors.

Everyone can be an exceptional patient, and the best time to start is before getting sick. Many people don't make full use of their life force until a near-fatal illness goads them into a "change of mind." But it doesn't have to be a last-minute awakening. The mind's power is available to us all the time, and it has more room to maneuver before disaster threatens. This process doesn't require allegiance to any particular religious belief or psychological system. Since cancer is the most common threatening disease in my practice, most of the experiences herein concern cancer, but the same principles apply to all diseases.

The fundamental problem most patients face is an inability to love themselves, having been unloved by others during some crucial part of their lives. This period is almost always childhood, when our relations with our parents establish our characteristic ways of reacting to stress. As adults we repeat these reactions and make ourselves vulnerable to illness, and our personalities often determine the specific nature of the illnesses. The ability to love oneself, combined with the ability to love life, fully accepting that it won't last forever, enables one to improve the quality of life. My role as a surgeon is to buy people time, during which they can heal themselves. I try to help them get well and at the same time to understand why they became sick. Then they can go on to true healing, not merely a reversal of one particular disease.

This book is a guide for such a transformation, as well as a record of my own education by my patients. I try to act as a conduit through which their painfully acquired talent for life can show you how to fight effectively for your own health. The book is not merely advice about what to do; that is plentiful. Rather it is a guide to the part of yourself that can choose your own best advice and then muster the will to follow it. I hope to reach beyond your rational mind, for miracles don't come from the cold intellect. They come from finding your authentic self and following what you feel is your own true course in life.

If you are suffering from some life-threatening disease, the change I'm talking about may save your life or prolong it well past medical expectations. At the very least it will enable you to get more out of your remaining time than you now think possible. If you have a minor disorder, or if you're not sick but not really enjoying life, the principles I've learned from exceptional patients can bring you joy and help you avoid illness in the future.

If you are a physician, I hope this book will give you some strategies for which you may have long felt a need, techniques that weren't covered in your education. Physicians rarely realize how differently they talk to cancer patients, compared with their other patients. We tell a heart-attack patient how to change his or her lifestyle—diet, exercise, and so on—thus offering hope that he or she can participate in getting well. But if the same patient were to put on makeup and a wig, then come back the next week and say, "I have cancer," most doctors would say, "If these treatments don't work, there's nothing else I can do for you." We must learn to give patients the option to participate in recovery from *any* type of disease.

I'm not using these pages to say, "I'm a better doctor than you." Rather I'm trying to explain why I felt like a failure until my patients taught me there's more to medicine than pills and incisions. I know your offices are filled with people who drain your energy and don't do well. I know the pain physicians feel. We have all of the problems other people have, as well as the one drummed into us in medical school: the role of mechanic-lifesaver, which defines illness and death as our failure. No one lives forever; therefore, death is not the issue. Life is. Death is not a failure. Not choosing to take on the challenge of life is. Let me show you the minority of patients who can restore your energy, the ones who get well even when they're not supposed to. Let me show you how to learn from your successful patients and help the others reawaken the "life wish" within. The process will inevitably help you heal yourself and make you a more successful healer.

We must remove the word "impossible" from our vocabulary. As David Ben-Gurion once observed in another context, "Anyone who doesn't believe in miracles is not a realist." Moreover, when we see how terms like "spontaneous remission" or "miracle" mislead and confuse us, then we will learn. Such terms imply that the patient must be lucky to be cured, but these healings occur through hard work. They are not acts of God. Remember that one generation's miracle may be another's scientific fact. Do not close your eyes to acts or events that are not always measurable. They happen by means of an inner energy available to all of us. That's why I prefer terms like "creative" or "self-induced" healing, which emphasize the patient's active role. Let me show you how exceptional patients work to heal themselves.

BERNIE S. SIEGEL, M.D.

New Haven, Conn.
April 1986

Kostoglotov [said], "All I'm saying is that we shouldn't behave like rabbits and put our complete trust in doctors. For instance, I'm reading this book." He picked up a large, open book from the window sill. "Abrikosov and Stryukov, *Pathological Anatomy,* medical school textbook. It says here that the link between the development of tumors and the central nervous system has so far been very little studied. And this link is an amazing thing! It's written here in so many words." He found the place. " 'It happens rarely, but there are cases of self-induced healing.' You see how it's worded? Not recovery through treatment, but actual healing. See?"

There was a stir throughout the ward. It was as though "self-induced healing" had fluttered out of the great open book like a rainbow-colored butterfly for everyone to see, and they all held up their foreheads and cheeks for its healing touch as it flew past.

"Self-induced," said Kostoglotov, laying aside his book. He waved his hands, fingers splayed. . . . "That means that suddenly for some unexplained reason the tumor starts off in the opposite direction! It gets smaller, resolves and finally disappears! See?"

They were all silent, gaping at the fairy tale. That a tumor, one's own tumor, the destructive tumor which had mangled one's whole life, should suddenly drain away, dry up and die by itself?

They were all silent, still holding their faces up to the butterfly. It was only the gloomy Podduyev who made his bed creak and, with a hopeless and obstinate expression on his face, croaked out, "I suppose for that you need to have . . . a clear conscience."

Aleksandr Solzhenitsyn, *Cancer Ward*

I

MINDING
THE
BODY

Love, Medicine, and Miracles is factually accurate, except that names, locales, and individual traits have been altered to preserve coherence while protecting privacy.

1

A new philosophy, a way of life, is not given for nothing. It has to be paid dearly for and only acquired with much patience and great effort.

—FYODOR DOSTOYEVSKY

The Privileged Listener

The idea of the exceptional patient is not taught in medical school. I came to it only after a long period of unhappiness and soul searching in my profession. I didn't have a class on healing and love, how to talk with patients, or the reasons for becoming a doctor. I was not healed during my training, and yet I was expected to heal others.

In the early 1970s, after more than a decade as a practicing surgeon, I was finding my job very painful. It wasn't a typical case of burnout; I could cope with the unending problems, the intensity of the work, and the constant life-or-death decisions. But I'd been trained to think my whole job was doing things to people in a mechanical way to make them better, to save their lives. This is how a doctor's success is defined. Since people often don't get better and since everyone eventually dies, I felt like a failure over and over again. Intuitively I felt there must be some way I could help the "hopeless" cases by going beyond my role as a mechanic, but it took years of difficult growth before I understood how to do so.

When I'd started out, I'd looked forward to facing new problems each day. It was an exciting challenge; it kept practice from becoming dull. After several years, however, the challenges themselves became monotonous. I would have loved an easy day when everything went according to schedule and I had only routine cases. But there were no "normal" days. It was only later that I became able to look upon the emergencies, and even the breakdowns in hospital procedure, as extra opportunities for helping people.

Surgeons aren't perfect. We always do our best, but complications still occur. Although disheartening, they keep us grounded and prevent us from starting to think of ourselves as gods. The one case that most shook my faith in myself was an injury to a facial nerve in a young girl I operated on early in my career. Seeing her wake up with half her face paralyzed made me want to hide forever. To become a surgeon in order to help people and then to end up disfiguring someone was a shattering experience. Unfortunately, I hadn't yet learned that my typical physician's response—to hide my pain when something went wrong—helped no one.

The pressure never let up. When a patient was taken to the operating room with severe bleeding, the staff was tense and panicky—until the surgeon walked in. Now the knot was in my stomach, and everyone else relaxed. There was no one to whom I could transfer it. I could only look inside myself for reassurance. As every operation began, the sweat poured off, and then, even though the lights were just as hot as before, I cooled off as things came under control. I used to feel desperately alone, expecting perfection of myself. The stress followed me home. Days before a difficult operation, I'd live it over and over in my mind, praying that the successful result I visualized would come to pass. Afterward, even if all went well, I'd suddenly wake up in the middle of the night questioning my decisions. Now, after years of being educated by my patients, I'm able to make each decision, live by it, and put it behind me, knowing I'm doing my best. Just like a minister who feels alone because he never learns to talk to God, a doctor feels alone if he or she never learns to talk with patients.

One of the worst hardships is having so little time to spend with one's family. The athlete can shower and go home after the game, but for doctors the working day often has no end. I had to adjust to the idea that being home on a weekend was a bonus, not something I could count on. Moreover, I was suffering from two-way guilt: snatching a few hours off felt like stealing time from my patients, while the sixteen-hour days felt like stealing time from my wife and children. I didn't know how to respond to the guilt or how to unify my life. Many nights I was too tired to enjoy my family after I did get home.

Once I was so exhausted that, when taking the babysitter home, I automatically drove to the hospital instead. She probably thought I was kidnapping her.

Even the time I managed to spend at home always seemed to get interrupted. The kids were constantly asking, "Are you on call tonight?" Everyone was nervous when I was on call, sure that the family evening wouldn't last. For most people the ringing of the telephone is a friendly sound. For us it meant anxiety and separation.

One of a physician's most unnerving trials is due to the fact that death comes in the middle of the night more often than at any other time, something I now understand. One can't help but feel a twinge of anger when a patient who has been in a coma for days passes away at 2 A.M., and the doctor and family must be awakened with the news. We think, "Why can't the dying have a little respect for the living?" Few of us ever mention this hostility. We just feel guilty about it. Then there's the added burden of having to be cheery and alert in the operating room at 7 A.M., despite family problems and two or three calls in the middle of the night.

On New Year's Day in 1974, I started keeping a journal. At first it was largely an outlet for my despair. "At times it seems the world is dying of cancer," I wrote one night. "Every abdomen you open is filled with it." And another night: "Your stomach hits the floor, and the horror sweeps over you as you see the future. How many faces must you look into and say, 'I'm sorry, it's an inoperable tumor'!"

I well remember Flora, one of my patients from that period. Her husband had recently died, and now she herself lay dying of uterine cancer, which two operations had failed to halt. She agonized over how much each day in the hospital cut into her life savings, which she had willed to her granddaughters. Wanting to prolong life, at the same time she wanted it to end so that no more of their education would be squandered on her frail body. "How," I wondered, "can I find strength to support all these people in their struggles?"

Thanks to the introspection of my diary I eventually realized I had to change my attitude toward medical practice. Throughout this period I was thinking seriously about finding another career. I considered becoming a teacher—or a veterinarian, because veterinarians can hug their patients. I couldn't decide what I wanted, but I realized that most of my choices had to do with people. Even in the painting I did as a hobby my only interest was portraits.

Then finally it dawned on me. Here I was, seeing a score of patients every day, as well as their families, dozens of doctors and nurses, and still I was looking for people. All this time I'd been dealing in cases, charts, diseases, remedies, staff, and prognoses, instead of people. I'd thought of my patients merely as machines I had to repair. I began to hear my co-workers' language in a new way. I remember addressing a conference of pediatricians that year. Many of them walked in late, excitedly explaining that an "interesting case"—a child nearing diabetic coma—had just been admitted. I realized with a shock what a distance that attitude put between the doctors and their "case," who happened to be a very sick, frightened child with distraught parents.

I became aware that, no matter how I'd struggled against it, I, too, had adopted this standard defense against pain and failure. Because I was hurting, I withdrew when patients needed me most. This became especially apparent when I returned from a long vacation in August 1974. For a few days I reacted only as a human being. Then I could feel the emotions slipping away and the professional veneer taking over. Yet I wanted to hang on to this sensitivity, because the coldness doesn't really save anyone from the pain. It just buries the hurt on a deeper level. I used to think a certain amount of this distancing was essential, but for most doctors I think it goes too far. Too often the pressure squeezes out our native compassion. The so-called detached concern we're taught is an absurdity. Instead, we need to be taught a rational concern, which allows the expression of feelings without impairing the ability to make decisions.

I was still debating whether to remain a surgeon or give up half a lifetime's learning to enter another specialty. I thought about psychiatry, in which I'd be able to help people without cutting into them. Then one of my cancer patients, a concert pianist named Mark, helped me realize that I could be happy without changing my profession. As his condition improved, all his friends told him he should go back to the stage, but he said he knew he didn't belong there anymore. He had found he was happier just playing the piano at home. He was still doing what he loved, but he had changed the context to suit his own needs. I realized I needed to do the same.

I tried to "step out from behind my desk" and open the door to my heart as well as my office. Now I literally have my desk against the wall so my patient and I are in position to face each other as equals. A telephone worker, a carpenter, and a medical student have said my office is all wrong because the desk isn't in the middle anymore. I had to explain that I want to see my patient with no obstacle between us, instead of relating as expert to failure.

I began encouraging my patients to call me by my first name. In the beginning it was quite scary to be just Bernie, not Dr. Siegel—to meet others as a person, not a label. It meant I had to like myself and deserve respect for what I did rather than what I'd learned in school. But the change was well worth it. It's a simple yet effective way to break down the barrier between doctor and patient.

Moving my desk and working on a first-name basis were only symptoms of a larger change. I committed the physician's cardinal sin: I "got involved" with my patients. For the first time I began to understand fully what it's like to live with cancer, knowing the fear that it may be spreading even while you talk to your doctor, do the dishes, play with the kids, work, sleep, or make love. How hard it is to keep one's integrity as a human being with this knowledge!

I no longer shielded myself emotionally from the scenes of sadness I had to witness each day. One day on rounds I found one patient lying on his side, drooling, his face stuporous from drugs, marshaling all his remaining concentration on holding his urinal, completely oblivious of a marvelous sunlit view through the window in front of him. He was lying in a pool of mingled grape juice and bile, and I found myself staring at the striking color of the stained sheet. The contrast of beauty and suffering overwhelmed me.

Soon, however, I found I could draw strength from my

patients. When I considered a man and wife, he with severe heart disease and she with widespread breast cancer, each trying to survive to help the other, my own sense of helplessness seemed somehow lessened. The compassion of another woman, in terrible pain from fractures of both arms but still worried that I was working too late, virtually banished my fatigue. When I said, "See you later," and a dying patient smiled and quipped, "I hope so," my sense of impending defeat faded, for I saw that the fear of death had not conquered that person's spirit. First I began hugging patients, figuring they needed my reassurance. Later I found I was saying, "*I need* to hug you," so that I could go on. And even if they were on respirators, my patients reached out to help me with a touch or a kiss, and my guilt, fatigue, and despair evaporated. They were saving me.

In the face of such courage, time and again I've wished I could do something to ease the passage. I began to feel that my profession's methods of attempting to prolong life and cure disease, among the noblest goals of our civilization, were sometimes crueler than the way of the wild, where serious illness is quickly relieved by death. It is said that one can never truly conceive of one's own death, but I'm sure some do when they must weigh the burden of the hours, days, or months remaining. The elderly often wonder why they have lived so long only to suffer such protracted misery and humiliation. I feel we should be able to do more to help a person let go and end life easily when the value of each day is gone. (I am talking about natural means of letting go, which are available to us all when death is not considered a failure.)

The need for compassion to balance our medical heroism never struck me more forcibly than during the death of Stephen, one of my partner's friends. After a massive heart attack, he was strapped to a bed, with tubes in every orifice. The damage was so great that a "no resuscitation" order was issued. He was weeping in pain and fear, but no one would authorize any painkillers, afraid that the drugs would hasten the inevitable and look like euthanasia. Finally my partner himself had to intercede, even though his friend was someone else's patient. He administered a shot of Nembutal. With the drug Stephen was able to relax and leave his body peacefully. He breathed a "Thank you" and slipped quietly away in five minutes. He would have been better off in the street than in the hospital. The end would have been quicker and less of an ordeal for all concerned. How can we say we're prolonging life when a person has become no more than a valve between the intravenous fluids going in and the urine coming out? All we're prolonging is dying. An editorial in the *Journal of the American Medical Association* entitled "Not on My Shift" expressed one doctor's dilemma in prolonging dying not extending life.

The word "hospital" comes from the Latin for "guest," but seldom is the institution truly hospitable. Little attention is given to caring or healing, as opposed to medicating. I've often wondered why designers couldn't at least make the ceilings pretty, since patients have to spend so much time staring at them. There's a TV in every room, but what music, what creative, meditative, or humorous video is available to help establish a healing environment? What freedom is given patients to maintain their identity?

Recently Sam, a patient who healed remarkably fast after a hernia repair, explained in a letter how a freer atmosphere helped him:

What *did* bother me, though, is why I was such a restrained, co-operative, model "good patient." I mean, I almost always make it known who I am wherever I go, making waves just to make waves.

So I gave it lots of thought, and the only answer I could come up with is that the hospital setting was so non-authoritative (especially with the new non-uniform dress code, which confused me) and the staff so *real*, that I had nothing to rebel against. And I think that my speedy healing, my *not* feeling helpless and dependent, made me feel *I* was in control anyway—and there was no need for me to make a big display of it.

While someone is in the hospital, the staff members become part of that person's family, for they see a patient more often and more intimately than anyone else. We must face that responsibility by offering the kind of loving support that we expect the family to provide. They can't do the whole job in a few hours of visiting time. I think of one of my patients, with carcinoma of the colon and metastases to the lungs and brain, refusing treatment so that he could die in the sun on his front porch, listening to the birds. Why can't hospitals be as warm?

By allowing myself to feel as sharply as I could the same pain and fear that my patients felt, I came to realize that there is an aspect of medicine more important than all the technical procedures. I learned that I had much more than surgery to offer and that my help could extend even to the dying and their survivors. In fact, I concluded that the *only* real reason to stay in this business was to offer people a friendship they can feel, just when they need it most. As my partner, Dick Selzer, who is a fine essayist as well as a fine surgeon, has written in *Mortal Lessons:*

I do not know when it was that I understood that it is precisely this hell in which we wage our lives that offers us the energy, the possibility to care for each other. A surgeon does not slip from his mother's womb with compassion smeared upon him like the drippings of his birth. It is much later that it comes. No easy shaft of grace this, but the cumulative murmuring of the numberless wounds he has dressed, the incisions he has made, all the sores and ulcers and cavities he has touched in order to heal. In the beginning it is barely audible, a whisper, as from many mouths. Slowly it gathers, rising from the streaming flesh until, at last, it is a pure *calling*—an exclusive sound, like the cry of certain solitary birds—telling that out of the resonance between the sick man and the one who tends him there may spring that profound courtesy that the religious call Love.

A GUIDE APPEARS

In June 1978, my practice of medicine changed as a result of an unexpected experience I had at a teaching seminar. Oncologist O. Carl Simonton and psychologist Stephanie Matthews (then his wife) gave a workshop—Psychological Factors, Stress, and Cancer—at the Elmcrest Institute in Portland, Connecticut. The Simontons were the first Western practitioners to use imaging techniques against cancer, and together with James L. Creighton they described their methods in *Getting Well Again*. The Simontons had already published their first results with "terminal" cancer patients. Of their first 159 patients, none of whom was expected to live more than a year, 19 percent had gotten rid of their cancer completely, and the disease was regressing in another 22 percent. Those who eventually did succumb had, on the average, doubled their predicted survival time.

When I looked around during the first workshop session, I was amazed and angered to find that I was the only "body doctor" there. There were a psychiatrist and a holistic practitioner, but not one other primary-care physician out of seventy-five participants. Those attending were mostly social workers, patients, and psychologists. I became even angrier when many of the participants told me they already knew about these techniques, because the things I was learning hadn't even been hinted at in my medical education. Here I was, an M.D., a *"M*edical *D*eity," and I didn't know what went on in the head at all! The literature on mind-body interaction was separate, and therefore unknown to specialists in other areas. I realized for the first time how far ahead theology, psychology, and holistic medicine are in this respect.

I thought about the health records of doctors. They have more problems with drugs and alcohol, and a higher suicide rate, than their patients. They feel more hopeless than their patients and die faster after the age of sixty-five. No wonder many people are reluctant to go to mainstream physicians. Would you take your car to a mechanic who couldn't get his own car to run?

The Simontons taught us how to meditate. At one point they led us in a directed meditation to find and meet an inner guide. I approached this exercise with all the skepticism one expects from a mechanistic doctor. Still, I sat down, closed my eyes, and followed directions. I didn't believe it would work, but if it did I expected to see Jesus or Moses. Who else would dare appear inside a surgeon's head?

Instead I met George, a bearded, long-haired young man wearing an immaculate flowing white gown and a skullcap. It was an incredible awakening for me, because I hadn't expected anything to happen. As the Simontons taught us to communicate with whomever we'd called up from our unconscious minds, I found that talking to George was like playing chess with myself, but without knowing what my alter ego's next move would be.

George was spontaneous, aware of my feelings, and an excellent adviser. He gave me honest answers, some of which I didn't like at first. I was still toying with the idea of a career change. When I told him, he explained that I was too proud to give up the hard-won technical proficiency of surgery and start from scratch in another discipline. Instead, he told me I could do more good by remaining a surgeon but changing my *self* to help my patients mobilize their mental powers against disease. I could combine the support and guidance of a minister or psychiatrist with the resources and expertise of a physician. I could practice "clergery," a term my wife coined. In the hospital I could be a role model for students, house officers, and even other physicians. George said, "You can go anywhere in the hospital. A clergyman or therapist can't. You are free to supplement medical treatment with love or death-and-dying counseling, in a way that nonphysicians are not."

I suppose you may call George a "meditatively released insight from my unconscious," or some such, if you must have an intellectual label for him. All I know is that he has been my invaluable companion ever since his first appearance. My life is much easier now, because he does the hard work.

George also helped me see things about medicine that I'd missed before. I saw that, as far as healing is concerned, exceptions do *not* prove the rule. If a "miracle," such as permanent remission of cancer, happens once, it is valid and must not be dismissed as a fluke. If one patient can do it, there's no reason others can't. I realized that medicine has been studying its failures when it should have been learning from its successes. We should be paying more attention to the exceptional patients, those who get well unexpectedly, instead of staring bleakly at all those who die in the usual pattern. In the words of René Dubos, "Sometimes the more measurable drives out the most important."

I began to see how reliance on statistics had warped my own thinking. Long ago I had operated on Jim, a patient with colon cancer. I told his family he had six months at most—this was back when I still predicted how long patients would live —but he proved me wrong. Several times he returned to me, and each time he walked in I'd think, "Aha! It's recurred at last," but it was always some minor unrelated problem. Every time I offered follow-up therapy for his cancer, he refused. He was too busy living and had no time for my treatments based on statistics. Jim has been healthy for well over a decade now.

At the other extreme are patients like Irving, a financial adviser who invested people's life savings according to statistics. He came to me with liver cancer. His oncologist told him what statistics said about his chances, and from then on he refused to fight for his life. He said, "I've spent my life making predictions based on statistics. Statistics tell me I'm supposed to die. If I don't die, my whole life doesn't make sense." And he went home and died.

One problem with cancer statistics is that most self-induced cures don't get into the medical literature. A survey of the reports on colorectal cancer found only seven such cases described between 1900 and 1966, although there have certainly been many more than that. A person who gets well when he isn't supposed to doesn't go back to his doctor. If he does, many doctors automatically assume his case was an error in diagnosis. In addition, most physicians consider such cases too "mystical" to submit to a journal, or think they don't apply to the rest of their patients, the "hopeless" ones.

Since I've changed my approach to focus on these rarities, however, I hear about "miraculous" healings everywhere I go. Once people realize that I know such things happen, they feel it's safe to tell me about them. After a talk at a local church, for example, a man handed me a card and whispered, "Read it later," and walked away. The handwritten note said:

Approximately 10 years ago your partner operated on my
dad and removed a section of his stomach. At this time you found
his entire lymph gland system to be cancerous. You advised me,
the oldest son, to inform the other members of my family of my

father's condition. I chose not to. Last Sunday my dad was surprised with a wonderful birthday party. He was 85 years old and my 80-year-old mom was smiling at his side!

I looked up the file, and, sure enough, we had considered this man's illness terminal over ten years before. He'd had cancer of the pancreas with lymph-node metastases. I reviewed the pathology slides, and there was no error in diagnosis. One physician's response to this case was "a slow-growing tumor." Today, this gentleman is 90. The tumor must be very slow-growing, indeed. In such cases physicians must learn to rush to the patient's home and ask why he didn't die when he was supposed to. Otherwise, such self-cures will not appear in the medical literature, and we will never learn from them that these are not instances of good luck, diagnostic errors, slow growing tumors, or well-behaved cancers.

A GROUP FOR RULE BREAKERS

After my experience with the Simontons, with the help of my wife, Bobbie, and Marcia Eager, then a nurse in my office, I started a therapy group called Exceptional Cancer Patients (ECaP) to help people mobilize their full resources against their disease. We adopted the Simontons' recently published *Getting Well Again* as a workbook and sent out a hundred letters to patients. The letter suggested we could help them live better and longer through the techniques ECaP would teach them. We expected hundreds of replies. We thought everyone who got a letter would tell several other cancer patients and bring them to the meeting. After all, I thought, doesn't everyone want to live? Don't many patients go to the ends of the earth for all sorts of alternative treatments that offer a glimmer of hope? I began to get nervous about how to handle the crowd that would appear.

Twelve people showed up.

That was when I started to learn, firsthand, what patients are really like. I found there are three kinds.

About 15 to 20 percent of all patients unconsciously, or

even consciously, wish to die. On some level they welcome cancer or another serious illness as a way to escape their problems through death or disease. These are the patients who show no signs of stress when they find out their diagnosis. As the doctor is struggling to get them well, they are resisting and trying to die. If you ask them how they are they say, "Fine." And what is troubling them? "Nothing."

One evening when I first began to understand this, I happened to be in the room as one of my partners was discussing treatment with Harold, a middle-aged colon-cancer patient, and his wife. I could hear his resistance to every option. Finally I broke in and said, "I don't think you really want to live."

His wife was enraged. But Harold himself spoke up. "Wait a minute," he said. "He's absolutely right. My father's ninety and senile and in a nursing home, and I never want to be like my father, so it's perfectly all right if I die of cancer now."

At that point the problem changed. It became a matter of getting him to feel that he could be in control of his life and death, to realize that he didn't have to give up many good years just to avoid the possibility of an unpleasant end. You don't have to be ninety and senile if you can say no to those who would artificially prolong your life—that is, your dying. After several days of discussing these issues and considering how he really felt about his life, Harold was able to go ahead with treatment for his cancer, and he is well today.

Not long afterward, a psychiatrist friend told me a story that brought home to me how far the death wish can go. He described one of his clients, a severely depressed man, who came in one day all smiles. The therapist asked what had happened, and the patient replied, "I don't need you anymore. I've got cancer now." When I think about such responses, I sometimes wonder what's the point of our search for longevity, when so many people feel so miserable and helpless that they don't want to live.

We must realize the pain most people suffer, and redefine our goals. What is healing? Is it a liver transplant or cure of an illness, or is it getting people to have peace of mind and live life to its fullest? I know quadriplegics who can say, "Fine," when asked, "How are you?"—because they have learned to love and give of themselves to the world. They are not denying their physical limits but rather transcending them.

In the middle of the spectrum of patients is the majority, about 60 to 70 percent. They are like actors auditioning for a part. They perform to satisfy the physician. They act the way they think the doctor wants them to act, hoping that then the doctor will do all the work and the medicine won't taste bad. They'll take their pills faithfully and show up for appointments. They'll do what they're told—unless the doctor suggests radical changes in their lifestyle—but it never occurs to them to question the doctor's decisions or strike out on their own by doing things for themselves that just "feel right." These are the people who, given a choice, would rather be operated on than actively work to get well.

At the other extreme are the 15 to 20 percent who are exceptional. They're not auditioning; they're being themselves. They refuse to play the victim. When acting out that role, patients cannot help themselves, for everything is being done *to* them.

I get many letters from groups called Aid to Cancer Victims, or some such title. The first thing I tell them is to change the group's name, because victims by definition do not have the control they need to redirect their mode of living. In our society, patients are automatically considered victims. Several years ago Herbert Howe, a former cancer patient and author of *Do Not Go Gentle,* appeared on ABC's *Good Morning, America* to tell how his disease disappeared after he quit standard medical therapy and took up exercise as an outlet for his anger. Even though he was free of cancer, his name appeared on the TV screen with the label "Cancer Victim."

Exceptional patients refuse to be victims. They educate themselves and become specialists in their own care. They question the doctor because they want to understand their treatment and participate in it. They demand dignity, personhood, and control, no matter what the course of the disease.

It takes courage to be exceptional. I remember one woman who, when told she had to go to the x-ray department, replied, "No. This test hasn't been explained to me." When the attendants told her, "You could die tonight if you don't have this test," she said, "Then I'll die tonight, but I'm not leaving my room." Immediately someone appeared to explain what the test was all about. Kathryn and Cornelius Ryan captured the exceptional patient's attitude in *A Private Battle,* an account of his battle with prostate cancer and eventual death from it in 1974. She wrote, "He went out like a tired lion, not a frightened lamb." It was the fatigue that finally made him let go. Fear was not the deciding factor.

Exceptional patients want to know every detail of their x-ray reports. They want to know what every number in their lab test printouts means. A doctor who harnesses that intense self-concern, instead of rejecting it and being "too busy," dramatically improves the patient's chances.

Physicians must realize that the patients they consider difficult or uncooperative are those who are most likely to get well. Psychologist Leonard Derogatis, in a study of thirty-five women with metastatic breast cancer, found that the long-term survivors had poor relationships with their physicians— as judged by the physicians. They asked a lot of questions and expressed their emotions freely. Likewise, National Cancer Institute psychologist Sandra Levy has shown that seriously ill breast-cancer patients who *expressed* high levels of depression, anxiety, and hostility survived longer than those who showed little distress. Levy and other researchers have also found that aggressive "bad" patients tend to have more killer T cells, white cells that seek and destroy cancer cells, than docile "good" patients. A group of London researchers under Keith Pettingale recently reported a ten-year survival rate of 75 percent among cancer patients who reacted to the diagnosis with a "fighting spirit," compared with a 22-percent survival rate among those who responded with "stoic acceptance" or feelings of helplessness or hopelessness.

To find out whether you have the outlook of an exceptional patient right now, ask yourself this question before reading further: Do you want to live to be a hundred? In ECaP we have found that the capacity to be an exceptional patient is accurately predicted by an immediate, visceral "Yes!" with no ifs, ands, or buts. Most people will say, "Well, yes, as long as you can guarantee I'll be healthy." However, the persons who become exceptional patients know that life comes with no such warranty. They willingly accept all the risks and challenges. As long as they're alive, they feel in control of their destiny, content to receive some happiness for themselves and give some to others. They have what psychologists call an *inner locus of control.* They do not fear the future or external events. They know that happiness is an inside job.

When I ask for a show of hands on this question, the response is invariably the same—about 15 to 20 percent—for an average audience. There are far fewer "Yes!" answers—only about 5 percent—in a roomful of doctors. Medical students are not so hopeless. It is trained into us. It's a tragedy that so few doctors have the self-confidence necessary to motivate others to believe in the future and care for themselves. Health-care providers are so used to seeing only illness and handicaps that they rarely have a positive attitude. When I go to a holistic health group or to a rustic area where self-reliant individuals live, almost all the hands go up. These are people who look to the future with confidence, knowing that respect and love are available at all ages.

I feel that all doctors should be required, as part of their training, to attend healing services, at which people with so-called incurable diseases appear. The physicians should be told they are not allowed to prescribe medications nor consider operations for these people, but simply told to go out and help them. Then doctors would learn that they can help by touching, praying, or simply sharing on an emotional level. It would also help to organize annual parties for survivors of serious illness, so that physicians could see and talk with their "successes," the people they've helped make well.

TEACHING EACH OTHER

The demands of exceptional patients and of ordinary ones are exactly analogous to the methods used by the doctors of slaves and of free men in ancient Greece, as described by Plato in Book IV of his *Laws:*

Did you ever observe that there are two classes of patients
. . . slaves and free men? And the slave-doctors run about and
cure the slaves or wait for them in dispensaries. Practitioners of
this sort never talk to their patients individually or let them talk
about their own individual complaints. The slave-doctor
prescribes what mere experience suggests, as if he had exact
knowledge; and when he has given his orders, like a tyrant, he
rushes off with equal assurance to some other servant who is ill.
. . . But the other doctor, who's a freeman, attends and practices
upon freemen; and he carries his enquiries far back, and goes into
the nature of the disorder; he enters into discourse with the
patient and with his friends, and is at once getting information
from the sick man, and also instructing him as far as he is able;
and he will not prescribe for him until he has first convinced him.
. . . If one of those empirical physicians, who practice medicine
without science, were to come upon the gentleman physician
talking to his gentleman patient and using the language almost of
philosophy, beginning at the beginning of the disease and
discoursing about the whole nature of the body, he would burst
into a hearty laugh. He would say what most of those who are
called doctors always have at their tongues' end: "Foolish fellow,"
he would say, "you are not healing the sick man, but educating
him; and he does not want to be made a doctor, but to get well."

Exceptional patients do indeed want to be educated and made
"doctors" of their own cases. One of the most important roles
they demand of their physicians is that of teacher.

As I began my transformation, people began to tell me
things I hadn't heard before. I learned what many doctors are
like in their offices. They shout. They keep patients waiting for
two hours but refuse them five minutes of discussion. A patient
told me that her former physician shouted, "There'll be only
one fucking cook in this kitchen," when challenged about the
choice of therapy. One physician scolded me for giving books
to his patient, a librarian with cancer. He said, "If you want me
to send you any more patients, you'll have to check everything
with me first." I told him I hadn't known the patient's mind
and body belonged to him. One patient told of walking into a
doctor's office and finding a sign on the desk that said, "Com-

promise means doing it my way." My advice is, if you see a sign like that, turn around and walk out.

At first I got furious at other doctors. My own anger was also intensified by the anger that ECaP group members had been holding in, but was safe to express in the group. Later I was able to get over my rage, as I understood how much pain many physicians bear in silence. I realized how the doctor's problems can be turned to a patient's advantage. As German poet Rainer Maria Rilke once wrote in reference to his own efforts to cheer up a young writer:

Do not believe that he who seeks to comfort you now lives untroubled among the simple and quiet words that sometimes do you good. His life has much difficulty and sadness and remains far behind yours. Were it otherwise he would never have been able to find those words.

As I began trying to teach my patients in the first ECaP group, I was amazed by the results. People whose conditions had been stable or deteriorating for a long time suddenly began to get well before my eyes. At first this made me very uncomfortable. I felt they were getting well for illegitimate reasons. Their progress had no obvious relation to drugs, radiation, or other traditional treatments. I felt like a charlatan or swindler and actually suggested disbanding the group.

At that point my patients had to explain to me what was going on. "We're getting better," they told me, "because you've given us hope and put us in control of our lives. You don't understand because you're a doctor. Sit and be patient." I did, and they became *my* teachers.

Then and there we adopted as our motto a sentence from the Simontons' book: "In the face of uncertainty, there is nothing wrong with hope." Some doctors have advised patients to stay away from me, so as not to build up "false hope." I say that in dealing with illness there is no such thing in a patient's mind. Hope is not statistical. It is physiological! The concepts of false hope and detached concern need to be discarded from the medical vocabulary. They are destructive for doctor and patient.

Whenever I work with medical students or other physicians, I ask them for a definition of false hope. They always hem
and haw, and fail to come up with one. I make it clear to them
that for most physicians "giving false hope" simply means telling a patient that he or she doesn't have to behave like a
statistic. If nine out of ten people with a certain disease are
expected to die of it, supposedly you're spreading "false hope"
unless you tell *all ten* they'll probably die. Instead, I say each
person could be the one who survives, because all hope is real
in a patient's mind.

Shlomo Breznitz, a psychologist at Hebrew University in
Jerusalem, recently demonstrated that positive and negative
expectation have opposite effects on blood levels of cortisol
and prolactin, two hormones important in activating the immune system. Breznitz had several groups of Israeli soldiers
make a grueling forced march of forty kilometers, but varied
the information he gave them. He told some they would march
sixty kilometers, but stopped them at forty, and told others
they would march thirty kilometers, then said they had another ten to go. Some were allowed to see distance markers,
and some had no clues as to how far they had walked or what
the total distance would be. Breznitz found that those with the
most accurate information weathered the march best, but the
stress hormone levels always reflected the soldiers' *estimates*
rather than the actual distance.

Even if what you most hope for—a complete cure—
doesn't come to pass, the hope itself can sustain you to accomplish many things in the meantime. Refusal to hope is nothing
more than a decision to die. I know there are people alive
today because I gave them hope and told them they didn't
have to die.

As I began to learn from my exceptional patients, I pro-
ceeded to make drastic changes in the way I practiced medicine. I was finally able to decide wholeheartedly to remain a
surgeon, so as to have direct, long-term relationships with patients, but I broadened my role from that of a mere mechanic
to include some of the functions of a preacher, teacher, and
healer. I accepted patients as individuals with choices and
options. We became a team.

A year before I began ECaP, I had shaved my head. Many associates thought it was a message of empathy with those who lose their hair during chemotherapy, but it had nothing to do with that. I later realized that it was a symbol of the uncovering that I was trying to make, baring my own emotions, spirituality, and love. In fact, one nurse reminded me that shaving the head is standard preparation for any operation on the brain.

The reactions were often revealing. Many people began to talk to me in a different way, as though I were handicapped. They shared their pain readily. Some physicians berated me for being different—all the more reason for keeping my new look.

My motives for baring my head became clearer at a workshop with Elisabeth Kübler-Ross. One of her techniques is to have participants make drawings illustrating aspects of their lives. I made a picture of a mountain with snow on top, drawn with white crayon on white paper. Below it was a pond with a fish out of water. The key was that something was being covered up (white on white), and the spiritual symbol (the fish) was out of place. I realized that what I meant to uncover was my love and spirituality, not my scalp. I had a wonderful dream that night, seeing myself with a full head of hair. After the workshop I told my family that I knew why I'd shaved my head and could now let my hair grow back, but our daughter Carolyn said, "No. It's easy to find you in the movies." Thus are great decisions made. My head remains bare, although Carolyn on occasion accidentally sits down next to other bald men.

It is from this period that I date my true career in healing, for it was only then that I found the full meaning of the work. The meaning consists of teaching patients how to live—teaching not from a pedestal but rather with the knowledge that *we teach what we want to learn.* Physicians must educate and at the same time learn from their patients. My endeavor to teach has been my own salvation, and I feel I am the greatest beneficiary of ECaP.

I became, as Bobbie phrased it, a "privileged listener." I began to hear all sorts of things that my patients felt were too emotional or too weird to tell other doctors. They told me about their dreams, premonitions, and self-diagnoses, the unorthodox things they'd like to add to their therapy, the so-called coincidences that give meaning to seemingly insignificant events, their feelings of love or fear or anger, the moments when they want to die.

A few years ago, for example, a woman named Mary came to see me after her consultation with one of my surgical associates. She asked, "Are you the one who does visualizing and all that stuff?" When I told her I was, she said, "Good. I want to tell you something. Somebody is with me all the time. He wears a white robe and a purple sash, and he has bad teeth. He's always in the room."

I asked her, "Well, what's his name? What does he have to say?"

She said, "I don't have the nerve to talk to him."

Mary was afraid to tell her family or her own doctor about her companion, for fear they'd think she was crazy, but once she thought I was a little weird, too, it was safe to tell me. Such openness is an enormous advantage for physicians. How can we hope to help people who can't tell us *everything* that's troubling them? What a relief to this woman to find out that her guest might be just a spontaneous version of my own guide, George!

Soon after we founded ECaP, some members of the group began to tell me that other physicians thought the things I was doing were crazy. By then, however, I was too happy about the members' improvement to care. I told them, "As long as you do well, I don't have to worry about my reputation."

One of the reasons other physicians feel leery of my methods is that they have not become privileged listeners. Sometimes they try to verify my work by asking a patient, "What's going on in your life?" The patient replies, "Nothing." They ask, "How are you feeling?" and the patient answers, "Fine." Then they wonder what I'm talking about.

Because so many patients have told me their innermost thoughts, I can now tell others, "I know the kinds of things that are going wrong in your life." Often I can suggest exactly what patients' emotional troubles are, based on the symptoms and location of their disease. Then they pour out their true feelings. After emergency surgery to remove several feet of dead intestine, a Jungian therapist recently told me, "I'm glad you're my surgeon. I've been undergoing teaching analysis. I couldn't handle all the shit that was coming up, or digest the crap in my life." Any connection with her feelings might not have occurred to another physician, but it was no coincidence to us that the intestines were the focal point of her illness. Recently after a mastectomy a woman said to me that she needed to get something off her chest.

I was tremendously excited after my first experiences with ECaP. I thought I was learning brand-new things that would revolutionize the practice of medicine overnight. I wrote a few articles about these discoveries, but the medical journals returned them. The editors said the subject matter was interesting but advised me to submit them to psychology journals. But psychologists didn't need this information. They already accepted the mind's role in disease. At about the same time I came across an article by Wallace C. Ellerbroek, formerly a surgeon, now a psychiatrist. The original subject of the piece had been the mind's role in cancer, but for seven years he couldn't get it published. He changed the focus to acne and it was printed in a major journal.

Next I tried presenting my experiences at medical meetings. The response was hard-nosed skepticism, if not outright scorn. Each discussion turned into a battle of wits, a game of "my statistics against yours." Almost no one was willing to admit, "Well, maybe there's something there. I'll try it." As a result, even though there is now plenty of scientific data to argue for psychotherapy in treatment of cancer and other diseases, I became convinced that statistics rarely alter deeply held beliefs. Numbers can be manipulated to make bias seem like logic. Rather than dwell on statistics, I now concentrate on individual experiences. To change the mind one must often speak to the heart . . . and listen. Beliefs are a matter of faith not logic.

Support is now coming my way and thinking is beginning to change. Studies are being done at Yale and elsewhere. As the politics of medicine change, funding for study changes, and new questions are explored.

2

*Medicine is not only a science, but also the art of
letting our own individuality interact with the
individuality of the patient.*

—ALBERT SCHWEITZER

The Healing Partnership

Mr. Wright, a client of psychologist Bruno Klopfer in 1957, had
far-advanced lymphosarcoma. All known treatments had become ineffective. Tumors the size of oranges littered his neck,
armpits, groin, chest, and abdomen. His spleen and liver were
enormously enlarged. The thoracic lymph duct was swollen
closed, and one to two quarts of milky liquid had to be drained
from his chest each day. He had to have oxygen to breathe, and
his only medicine now was a sedative to help him on his way.

Despite his state, Mr. Wright still had hope. He'd heard of
a new drug called Krebiozen, which was to be evaluated at the
clinic where he lay. He didn't qualify for the program, because
the experimenters wanted subjects with a life expectancy of at
least three and preferably six months. Wright begged so hard,
however, that Klopfer decided to give him one injection on
Friday, thinking he would be dead by Monday and the
Krebiozen could be given to someone else. Klopfer was in for
a surprise:

I had left him febrile, gasping for air, completely bedridden.
Now, here he was, walking around the ward, chatting happily
with the nurses, and spreading his message of good cheer to any
who would listen. Immediately I hastened to see the others. . . .
No change, or change for the worse was noted. Only in Mr.
Wright was there brilliant improvement. The tumor masses had
melted like snowballs on a hot stove, and in only these few days,
they were half their original size! This is, of course, far more
rapid regression than most radio-sensitive tumors could display
under heavy X-ray given every day. And we already knew his

tumors were no longer sensitive to irradiation. Also, he had had no other treatment outside of the single useless "shot."

This phenomenon demanded an explanation, but not only that, it almost insisted that we open our minds to learn, rather than try to explain. So, the injections were given three times weekly as planned, much to the joy of the patient. . . . Within 10 days he was able to be discharged from his "deathbed," practically all signs of his disease having vanished in this short time. Incredible as it sounds, this "terminal" patient gasping his last breath through an oxygen mask was now not only breathing normally, and fully active, he took off in his own plane and flew at 12,000 feet with no discomfort.

. . .[W]ithin two months, conflicting reports began to appear in the news, all of the testing clinics reporting no results. . . . This disturbed Mr. Wright considerably. . . . [H]e was . . . logical and scientific in his thinking, and he began to lose faith in his last hope. . . . [A]fter two months of practically perfect health, he relapsed to his original state and became very gloomy and miserable.

But Klopfer saw an opportunity to explore what was really going on—to find out, as he put it, how quacks achieve some of their well-documented cures. (Remember all healing is scientific.) He told Wright that Krebiozen really was as promising as it had seemed, but that the early shipments had deteriorated rapidly in the bottles. He told of a new superrefined, double-strength product due to arrive tomorrow.

The news came as a great revelation to him, and Mr. Wright, ill as he was, became his optimistic self again, eager to start over. By delaying a couple of days before the "shipment" arrived, his anticipation of salvation had reached a tremendous pitch. When I announced that the new series of injections were about to begin, he was almost ecstatic and his faith was very strong.

With much fanfare, and putting on quite an act . . . I administered the first injection of the doubly potent, fresh preparation—consisting of *fresh water* and nothing more. The results of this experiment were quite unbelievable to us at the time, although we must have had some suspicion of the remotely possible outcome to have even attempted it at all.

Recovery from the second near-terminal state was even more

dramatic than the first. Tumor masses melted, chest fluid vanished, he became ambulatory, and even went back to flying again. At this time he was certainly the picture of health. The water injections were continued, since they worked such wonders. He then remained symptom-free for over two months. At this time the final AMA announcement appeared in the press —"Nationwide tests show Krebiozen to be a worthless drug in treatment of cancer."

Within a few days of this report Mr. Wright was readmitted to the hospital in extremis; his faith was now gone, his last hope vanished, and he succumbed in less than two days.

One of the best ways to make something happen is to predict it. Pooh-poohed for some twenty years by the medical establishment, the placebo effect—the fact that about one-fourth to one-third of patients will show improvement if they merely *believe* they are taking an effective medicine even if the pill they are taking has no active ingredient—has now been accepted as genuine by most of the profession.

Dr. Howard Brody of Michigan State asserts that a positive placebo response occurs when three factors are optimally present: the meaning of the illness experience for the patient is altered in a positive manner; the patient is supported by a caring group; and the patient's sense of mastery and control over the illness is enhanced. Nearly all so-called primitive medicine uses the placebo factor via rituals that foster assurance in the healing force, whether it is defined as an external god or an internal energy. Faith healing relies on the patient's belief in a higher power and the healer's ability to act as a channel to it. Sometimes a mere artifact or saint's relic is conduit enough. For a believer a bottle labeled Lourdes Holy Water has healing properties even if there's only tap water in it. Thus Christian Scientists sometimes succeed ·in healing themselves because they're taught to seek peace of mind and give themselves up to a higher power. This is why it's so important that a physician have a good reputation as a "mechanic" and the ability to project confidence. A patient's hope and trust lead to a "letting go" that counteracts stress and is often the key to getting well.

Unfortunately, peace often does not come until death is near. That is when people can let go. I see many patients close to death who are still worried about the electric bill and children staying out too late. If I tell them, "Let go of all that and have a nice day—it may be your last day on earth," the next morning I find them feeling better and eating a big breakfast. When I ask what happened, they say, "I took your advice."

HOPE THROUGH TRUST

"Primitive" medicine is actually much more sophisticated than ours in the use of the mind, perhaps because it has fewer drugs that are effective without help from the placebo effect. Robert Müller, Assistant Secretary-General of the United Nations and author of *Most of All They Taught Me Happiness,* has written of an African delegate who had been told by a New York doctor that he had cancer and would die within a year. The delegate told Müller and his other friends that he was going home to die but would ask his relatives to notify them of the funeral so they could attend. Eighteen months went by. Having no word, Müller, presuming the delegate dead, called his home village to learn the details. He was pleasantly surprised to hear the man himself, sounding quite robust.

Soon after his return home, the delegate explained, the local witch doctor had come to him and said, "You look depressed." When he learned why, he told the sick man to come to his hut the next day.

The witch doctor began therapy with a simple symbolic gesture. From a large cauldron he dipped a small cup of liquid and said, "This cup represents the part of your brain you are using. The cauldron the rest. I will teach you to use the rest." Today the man is alive and well.

I am not urging that Western technological medicine be abandoned for earlier kinds, but I am asking that we become open to the healing gift within us. Over and over, psychologists remind us that most of us use only about 10 percent of our mind's capacity. Let us then, as the witch doctor taught, use the other 90 percent. Science teaches that we must see in order to believe, but we must also believe in order to see. We must be receptive to possibilities that science has not yet grasped, or we will miss them. It's absurd not to use treatments that work, just because we don't yet understand them.

Open-mindedness is the hallmark of all physicians who are truly interested in helping their patients. For many years, Dr. William S. Sadler, one of the leading proponents of drug-based medicine at the turn of the century, studied "mind cures," as they were then called. In the introduction to a series of articles in the *Ladies' Home Journal* in August 1911, he wrote:

I used to have a popular lecture showing the follies of these "cures," but I observed that I never made a convert from the psychic ranks. And all this time some of these systems went on curing patients that I hadn't cured and couldn't cure.

Sadler opened his mind, made a thorough inquiry into the subject, and came away convinced that the power of suggestion, while not a panacea, was a worthy ally of pharmacy, surgery, and hygiene.

The placebo effect depends on a patient's trust in the physician. I've become convinced that this relationship is more important, in the long run, than any medicine or procedure. Psychiatrist Jerome Frank of Johns Hopkins University found evidence for this belief in a 1969 study by R. C. Mason, G. Clark, R. B. Reeves, and B. Wagner of ninety-eight patients who had surgery for detached retinas. The subjects' independence, optimism, and faith in their doctors before the operations were assessed. The patients with a high level of trust healed faster than the others.

To create a relationship of trust the doctor and patient must learn each other's beliefs. A doctor's confidence in a certain treatment can be negated by a patient's unspoken rejection of it. This is why I study patients' drawings and dreams to learn unacknowledged feelings about therapy. Otherwise, I may choose what I think is a wonderful treatment, yet encounter every conceivable side effect, so therapy must be stopped. The patient may not have wanted this therapy from the first but didn't have the courage to tell me, or may be rejecting it at an unconscious level. However, if I have a drawing showing that the patient perceives the treatment as a poison or injurious, we can proceed from that point. We can try to modify the patient's attitude toward the treatment or choose a different form of therapy. A positive drawing done by a fearful patient may also help allay fears and allow therapy to commence.

The belief systems of physicians and patients interact, but patients' bodies respond directly to their own beliefs, not their doctors'. Physicians tend to be more logical, statistical, and rigid, and less inclined to have hope, than their patients. When physicians run out of remedies, they're likely to give up. They must realize, however, that lack of faith in the patient's ability to heal can severely limit that ability. We should never say, "There's nothing more I can do for you." There's always something more we can do, even if it's only to sit down, talk, and help the patient hope and pray.

The usual attitude of doctors is summed up perfectly in the experience of Stephanie, one of our ECaP patients. After the diagnosis of cancer, her doctor outlined the rest of her life, as predicted by statistics, right into an early grave. She asked what she could do, and he told her, "All you've got is a hope and a prayer." She asked, "How do I hope and pray?" He replied, "I don't know. It's not my line." Her ECaP experience taught her how to hope and pray, and Stephanie has altered the course of her disease, exceeding expectations, and her doctor is now making notes about her success. Later she wrote that this doctor, in mentioning hope and prayer, "was actually prescribing the one medication that was going to cure me, *and he never even knew it.*"

The reverse effect can even kill. Frances, a woman in her eighties, came to me when she lost faith in her former physician because of his negative attitude. Despondent because of repeated nagging illnesses, she reached out to him for reassurance, and he asked her, "Well, how long do you want to live, anyway?" She was smart enough to see what this outlook was doing to her, and she left.

I remember one man who wasn't so lucky. Ellen, an ECaP group member, once called her husband, Ray, who was hospitalized with cancer, to see how he felt. He said, "Fine." Fifteen minutes later she arrived for a visit, and he was dead. In the interim, Ray, who'd been in and out of the hospital several times, had asked his doctor when he'd be able to leave. After the reply, "Oh, I don't think you'll make it this time," he died within minutes.

The physician's habitual prognosis of how much time a patient has left is a terrible mistake. It's a self-fulfilling prophecy. It must be resisted even though many patients keep asking, "How long? How long?" They want someone else to define the limits of life instead of taking part in that determination themselves. People who like their doctors and who are passive often die right on schedule, as though to prove them right.

Physicians must stop letting statistics determine their beliefs. Statistics are important when one is choosing the best therapy for a certain illness, but once that choice is made, they no longer apply to the individual. All patients must be accorded the conviction that they *can* get well, no matter what the odds.

Exceptional patients have the ability to throw statistics aside—to say, "I can be a survivor"—even when the doctor isn't wise enough to do so. Just think of the courage it took for someone to conquer a certain type of cancer that no one had ever conquered before. Hope instilled that kind of courage in William Calderon, who achieved the first documented recovery from Acquired Immune Deficiency Syndrome (AIDS).* Calderon was diagnosed in December 1982. His doctors told him he would probably be dead in six months. Understandably, he became depressed and hopeless. Almost immediately Kaposi's sarcoma, the type of cancer that most often accompanies AIDS, appeared and began spreading rapidly on all areas of his skin and throughout his gastrointestinal tract.

Soon Judith Skutch, co-founder with astronaut Edgar Mitchell of the Institute of Noetic Sciences and now President of the Foundation for Inner Peace, arrived at Calderon's hairstyling salon for her regular appointment. Noticing by his eyes that he had been weeping, she got him to tell her the reason.

*Calderon's case is discussed at length by Jean Shinoda Bolen, M.D., in the March/April 1985 issue of *New Realities*, pp. 9–15.

Her next words turned out to be the key to saving his life. She said, "William, you don't have to die. You can get well."

Skutch described the Simontons' work with cancer patients. With unwavering love and support from her and from his lover, Calderon came to believe in his own survival. By continuing at the job he loved, he refused to give in to the disease. Instead he began meditating and using mental imagery to combat it. He worked to restore strained relationships with his family and achieved peace of mind by forgiving people he felt had hurt him. He loved his body with exercise, good nutrition, and vitamin supplements. And from that point on his immune system showed increased response and his tumors began to shrink. Two years after the diagnosis, Calderon showed no signs of AIDS.

The exceptional patient often gets angry at a doctor's heavy-handed pronouncement of doom. Linda, a nurse I know who refused chemotherapy, was told by her M.D., "You'll be sorry. You'll come crawling back here in six months." She kept thinking, "That S.O.B.! I won't die, just to prove he's wrong." She lived for over five years without his therapy, and then decided to use it to live even longer.

I have a copy of a letter from a young woman named Louise to a "rock 'n' roll doctor," who had a radio show combining music with medical advice and with whom she became close friends while she was in the hospital. As a teenager Louise developed cancer of the ovary with metastases to the lungs and abdomen. Her oncologist "gave" her six to twelve months to live with chemotherapy. She told him only God could decide when her number was up, and began to take her life into her own hands. She left home because of stressful living conditions there, got her own apartment, and spent her last ten dollars to place a newspaper ad, looking for other cancer patients who needed her help. At one point her oncologist had refused her any further treatment because she was "too far gone," but six months after she had taken the path of her own choosing, all her tumors had disappeared. Her doctor couldn't even tell her this out loud. Instead, with tears in his eyes, he handed her a prescription form on which he'd written, "Your cancer has disappeared." On the day she was supposed to be dead, Louise sent him a joking note asking, "Where should I send the casket?"

The "rock 'n' roll doctor" wrote to tell me that, if he hadn't happened to hear me speak about exceptional patients, he probably wouldn't have made the connection between Louise's "miraculous" recovery and her spiritual growth. Instead, it made sense to him, and they both came to one of our ECaP meetings to share the experience.

Louise chose to love and give, making the kind of spiritual and psychological changes that people who experience self-induced healings always make. It takes enormous strength to do this when the voice of authority is telling you you're supposed to die. The problem is, exceptional patients are a minority. If eight out of ten patients are not survivors, it's easy to ignore the two who potentially are.

I'm trying to publicize such cases so that more doctors look for them among their own patients. Then they will see that healing is not a coincidence. When so defined, as in the phrase "spontaneous remission," it teaches doctors nothing and stimulates no inquiry into the causes behind it. On the contrary, healing is a creative act, calling for all the hard work and dedication needed for other forms of creativity.

I often get letters from doctors about patients I've referred. When a doctor reports amazing improvements in a patient's condition, he or she almost never mentions that person's beliefs and lifestyle, but when I inquire, I find the patient *always* has made some drastic change toward a more loving and accepting outlook. The patient seldom tells an unreceptive doctor about this, however.

Unexpected healing happens often enough that physicians must learn to project hope at all times, even in what seem to be the final hours. Patients are not looking for the results of a medical Gallup poll. They're looking for a success-oriented relationship. They're looking for someone to say, "Hold on, you can make it. We'll help you"—as long as the patient wants to stay alive. It is not for us to evaluate the worth of continued life for another person. As long as my patients are living in a way that has value to *them,* I'm there to help them continue.

However, if a patient has decided it's time to die, I see no contradiction in aiding with that, too. I can help resolve conflicts that drain energy, knowing that this resolution may initiate healing after all. Thus, although telling people they will die by such and such a day is destructive and has no place in medical practice, acceptance of death need not take away hope. Paradoxically, preparation for death can promote the cause of life. One cancer patient, for example, was looking awful one Friday, and told me she wanted to die. I said, "Tell your children and your parents how you feel, and then it's okay. They don't realize how bad you feel." On Monday when I returned to the hospital, she looked great; she was wearing her wig, a suit, and makeup. I said "What happened?" She said, "I told my parents how I felt and my kids how I felt, and then I felt so good I didn't want to die." And she was discharged from the hospital.

Despite the need for optimism, no part of the diagnosis should ever be hidden. The truth can always be delivered with hope, since no one can be certain of the future. Moreover, I can now accept illness and see my primary task as helping patients achieve peace of mind. This puts the physical problems in perspective. Getting well is not the only goal. Even more important is learning to live without fear, to be at peace with life, and ultimately death. Then healing can occur and one is no longer set up for failure (by believing one can cure all physical problems and never die).

Twenty years ago "benign deception" was common. Since then, attitudes have undergone a complete about-face. A 1979 survey by Dr. Dennis Novack and his co-workers, published in the *Journal of the American Medical Association,* found that 97 percent of doctors preferred to tell cancer patients their diagnosis, as compared with 90 percent who said they would *not* in a survey two decades earlier.

Fortunately, clinicians have realized that patients usually know the truth anyway. On an unconscious and even on a conscious level, patients know what is going on in their bodies. Bill, a physician patient of mine, had difficulty swallowing at dinner one night. He said he knew he had cancer, because his father had cancer of the esophagus and stomach at the same age. One symptom and he *knew*. Of course, everyone reassured him, but tests proved him right.

Lies and evasions drive families apart just when they most need to be united in facing the crisis honestly. Families often say, "Don't tell mama. She can't handle it." When I ask mama what she thinks is wrong, she says, "I guess it's cancer." The word is out then, and we can talk about what cancer means to the family—a challenge or a death sentence. Deceit also drives out confidence. When the physician hesitates, cannot pronounce the word "cancer," or puts on a false front, the patient's mind immediately translates: "The doctor can't handle this. There is no hope."

Too many doctors today have gone from benign deception to a brutal honesty that also does more harm than good. I recently received a heartrending letter from a patient's wife, explaining that her husband would not be keeping his second appointment with me because he had committed suicide.

It was two days after he was told—with the most careless brutality—that he would never play tennis, captain a boat, or go to work again, all—particularly the first two—things he loved.

All along, he had had the most innocent faith in his doctors, not that they could effect a cure, but that they were doing their best. They, particularly his oncologist, had no best.

Far better to admit that the situation is grave, yet to remind the patient in truth that there is no "incurable" disease from which someone has not recovered, even at the threshold of death.

When a doctor can instill some measure of hope, the healing process sometimes starts even before treatment begins. I recall one of my patients whose radiologist told her that the drugs were working, because her bone scan had improved dramatically. She replied, "If you'll look at my schedule, you'll see I haven't started chemotherapy yet. It must be that shiny-headed doctor."

Dr. Alexandra Levine, a California oncologist, recently received a grant to study psychosocial aspects of cancer. She applied for it because of a similar experience. A man with extensive lymphoma was brought to her office. The patient's wife insisted he visit her before traveling all the way to Germany for a "miracle" cure he wanted to try. When Dr. Levine saw the panic in the man's eyes, she spent an hour simply calming and reassuring him. When he came back the next week, his tumors had shrunk by about half. She said, "I wish I had started your treatment last week." He told her, "You did."

Hope comes about largely as a result of the patient's confidence and trust in the healer. This bond is forged in many ways. Certain essentials—compassion, acceptance, availability, a willingness to provide information—are obvious. That is why preoperative visits by the surgical team are so important. They not only help the patient through the surgery but also speed recovery. In a study described in Dr. Herbert Benson's *The Mind/Body Effect*, a group led by Dr. Lawrence Egbert at Harvard showed that patients who received a visit from the anesthesiologist the night before surgery, as well as other explanations and reassurances not given to a group of control patients, needed only half as much pain medication. They also left the hospital more than two and a half days sooner, on the average, than the control group.

A sense of humor is an enormous asset, too. Many times when I'm in a room with a "dying" patient we are laughing. Out in the hallway, the other staff members often think we are denying reality. We're simply still alive and thus able to laugh. Hospital personnel must realize that people aren't "living" or "dying." They are either alive or dead. As long as they are alive, we must treat them that way. I find the word "terminal" terribly upsetting. It means we've begun to treat that person as though he or she were already dead. Studies have shown that it takes doctors and nurses longer to respond to the call button from a "terminal" patient's room than a button pressed by someone who is not labeled that way. The word implies a state of mind more than a physical condition, and it turns off the staff's empathy and ability to give the full measure of care needed. It also confronts them with their own mortality.

It's also essential that patients know they can express

anger to their physician without hurting the relationship. I've often heard people complain about their doctors, only to be asked not to mention it to them for fear of retribution in the future. Unexpressed anger hurts the patient and must be shared to establish a healing team. How poor the bond must be for a patient to believe that a doctor would not respond to criticism on a professional level. I'm happy when patients express anger at me, because it means they feel safe with me, that we have a good relationship and they are behaving like survivors.

My father had surgery several years ago and was sent home with what I thought were very poor instructions. As a result, he suffered complications. I wrote to each physician, the surgeon and the internist, expressing my feelings. From the surgeon I got a letter blaming me for the problems. The internist wrote back saying, "Thank you. Every now and then we need a letter like that to help us do our best." I advised my father, "Change surgeons and keep your internist."

UNCONSCIOUS AWARENESS

Because of its effect on the patient, a doctor's attitude is often crucial to the success of treatment. One of the most important factors is a patient's confidence in having the doctor's undivided attention. I remember being in an operating room as an intern years ago with a patient under spinal anesthesia. Hearing only sports talk among the staff, he asked plaintively, "Won't someone please say something about me and my operation?" Picture the absurdity of a person with severe cancer having to listen to a technician worry about missing a hockey game or a doctor complain about being late to have her hair done. Only empathy can build the connection needed for healing. When a doctor sits down for one minute at the bedside to talk, the patient experiences it as five or ten minutes. If the doctor stands in the doorway, the same visit seems like fifteen seconds.

Attitude counts even when the patient is unconscious, asleep, in coma, or under anesthesia. Milton Erickson, the great psychiatrist and hypnotherapist, showed in the early 1950s that voices known and meaningful to the patient were heard and understood during anesthesia. A Baltimore obstetrician once told me he had noticed a subtle change in his patients' behavior many years ago when the switch was made from ether to lighter anesthetics. To investigate, he brought a court stenographer into the operating room to record every word spoken during several caesarean sections. He found that under hypnosis these patients could repeat the conversations word for word.

Recent work has confirmed this unconscious awareness. Henry Bennett, a psychologist at the University of California Medical School at Davis, played a tape to anesthetized patients asking them to signal that they had heard the message by touching their ears during a post-op interview. Nearly all of them repeatedly tugged at their ears without being aware of it, but none could remember the message. In another experiment, Dr. Bennett asked unconscious patients to make one hand warmer than the other, and they promptly complied. With another group of patients, nonhypnotic pre-op suggestions that blood would leave the hip area reduced blood loss by half during hip surgery. We have incredible mechanisms by which we can direct chemotherapy to a cancer or divert blood and starve a tumor.

For years I've been utilizing the ability of unconscious patients to hear. I talk to persons in coma to let them know their medical status. In one case I told a woman who had been in coma for three years, with no signs of recovery, that her family was giving her permission to go, and that by dying she would not be a failure as a mother. I said they would miss her, but it was all right to let go if she wanted to. In fifteen minutes she died. When I enter a room where a patient is sleeping, I simply announce myself softly and let his unconscious awareness awaken him if he wants to talk to me at that moment. If he doesn't wake up and there's no urgent problem, I return later.

Several surgeons have now begun using the anesthetized mind's powers to help prevent complications. After lower back surgery, many people have trouble urinating and often need catheters because of spasms in the pelvic muscles. One group of researchers suggested to patients on the operating table that they would be able to relax the crucial muscles afterward. None of these patients needed catheters.

In the operating room I'm constantly communicating with patients about what is happening, and I've found that this can make the difference between life and death. Talking reassuringly to patients who are having cardiac irregularities during surgery can reverse the irregularities or slow a rapid pulse. Recently I was operating on a very husky young man, built like a football player. His size led to some minor technical problems, and while solving them I looked up at the monitor and saw that his pulse was 130. I knew that he had been anxious about the operation, so I said to him, "Victor, I'm having some mechanical difficulties because you're a big guy, but there's no problem with the surgery. This part is just a little difficult to do. You're doing well. Don't be nervous. I'd like your pulse to be 83." During the next few minutes, without any other medication, his pulse came right down to 83 and remained there. Many anesthesiologists who've heard of such episodes have begun speaking to their anesthetized patients, giving them calming messages. Fear filled messages can increase the incidence of cardiac arrest.

Once, as I finished a difficult emergency abdominal operation on a young, very obese man, his heart stopped just as we were about to move him to the recovery room. He didn't respond to resuscitation. The anesthesiologist had given up and was walking out the door when I spoke out loud into the room, "Harry, it's not your time. Come on back." At once the cardiogram began to show electrical activity, and the man ultimately recovered fully. I can't prove it, of course, but I am sure the verbal message made the difference. I know the experience made believers out of the other staff members who were present, and there is certainly no reason *not* to communicate with a patient in every possible way.

It's especially important to avoid negative messages, because the anesthetized patient's conscious defense mechanisms aren't functioning. Recently a medical student named Tim wrote me a letter describing one surgeon's operating-room manner:

I heard the surgeon talking with a vengeance in his voice that I thought was reserved solely for medical students. "This lady," he proclaimed, "tells me she's holistic! Hoooolistic, ha! She's so holistic that the highlight of her life was probably buying a bird-watching book!" Soon after, I heard, "She's so holistic that she thinks that radiation will hurt her. Why, she's uglier than the secretary on the Beverly Hillbillies." On and on it went, insult after insult, as if she was a thousand miles away and not under general anesthesia three feet from where he spoke. "She says she's hypoglycemic. Ha! She's a *strange* woman."

Then he announced, "Look at this. This is cancer. It's full of cancer, it's malignant," and he pulled out a chunk of tissue as though he were cutting a piece of his favorite apple pie.

Needless to say, she awoke from anesthesia cold, crying, and in lots of pain.

Tim befriended the woman through further tests and a radical mastectomy, playing one of my ECaP tapes for her. His love helped her take more control over her treatment, which in turn reduced her pain. She refused radiation and chemotherapy, which she feared as poisonous, in favor of the holistic alternatives she believed in. In his letter, Tim noted that it's too early to know the outcome of her illness, but he met her soon after her discharge from the hospital and found her vibrant, energetic, and glowing with love.

She also cleared up a mystery that had been puzzling Tim for several days. The same surgeon who had been so abusive had performed her mastectomy, but that time he was caring and gentle. Tim wrote:

Why did he visit her in the recovery room and call her at home? Why was he the only member of the hospital staff to support her decision to refuse further testing, telling her to "go home, rest, and get healthy"?

It seems that on the morning of surgery as he made his fifteen-second preoperative visits, she caught him off guard with a hug like he'd never experienced before (at least not from any of his patients). At first he was taken aback, not knowing how to respond. Later he hugged her back, and they both strongly embraced.

Sometimes it's not clear who is the patient and who is the physician. I don't know if either of them has cured their cancers, but they have helped each other.

I always make sure that operating-room personnel don't say anything they wouldn't say if the patient were awake. When a surgeon makes a quip like, "If he ever leaves here, it'll be feet first," it's no wonder the patient wakes up crying in the recovery room. One can be honest about the diagnosis and still implant positive thoughts about the future treatment. A simple statement like "You'll wake up comfortable, thirsty, and hungry"—modified for obese patients—will promote recovery. Even the desire to smoke can be reduced by a suggestion at the end of the operation. I also do not hesitate to ask the patient not to bleed if circumstances call for it. It's well known that yogis and hypnotized subjects can control bleeding, and the verbal request also seems to work during anesthesia. I sometimes wonder if anesthesia suggestions might sometimes be utilized as a form of psychotherapy.

The ambience of the clinical environment influences the attitude of both doctor and patient. I fear that we lost one of our most important sources of strength—a connection to God and nature—when hospital planners took the windows out. A view of the outside world reminds us of our link to all life, helping us survive. Recent research at a hospital in Pennsylvania showed that patients whose rooms faced an open courtyard, a tree, and the sky got well faster than those whose rooms faced a brick wall. In *Mortal Lessons* Dick Selzer has written eloquently of the same effect from the physician's viewpoint:

Not long ago, operating rooms had windows. It was a boon and a blessing in spite of the occasional fly that managed to strain through the screens and threaten our very sterility. For the adventurous insect drawn to such a ravishing spectacle, a quick swat and, Presto! The door to the next world sprang open. But for us who battled on, there was the benediction of the sky, the applause and reproach of thunder. A Divine consultation crackled in on the lightning! And at night, in Emergency, there was the pomp, the longevity of the stars to deflate a surgeon's ego. It did no patient a disservice to have Heaven looking over his doctor's shoulder. I very much fear that, having bricked up our windows, we have lost more than the breeze; we have severed a celestial connection.

◆ ◆ ◆

To work in windowless rooms is to live in a jungle where you cannot see the sky. Because there is no sky to see, there is no grand vision of God. Instead, there are the numberless fragmented spirits that lurk behind leaves, beneath streams. The one is no better than the other, no worse. Still, a man is entitled to the temple of his preference. Mine lies out on a prairie, wondering up at Heaven. Or in a many windowed operating room where, just outside the panes of glass, cows graze, and the stars shine down upon my carpentry.

To reestablish this celestial connection I use music, whose healing properties have been known since biblical times. During the age of the prophets, harp players would perform special pieces of music to provoke a mental state in which extrasensory powers were thought to be activated, as is said of Elisha—"And it came to pass, when the minstrel played, that the hand of the Lord came upon him." David played for King Saul to help him recover from his depression and paranoia.

Music opens a spiritual window. When I first brought a tape recorder into the O.R., it was considered an explosion hazard. But we ran it on batteries, and then the nurses and anesthesiologists felt so much better that, if I forgot my music, they'd ask for it. Now there are tape recorders in almost all the operating rooms in New Haven.

A recent study at the Pacific Medical Center of Presbyterian Hospital in San Francisco showed that music eased anxiety, stress, and pain in children and adults during the traumatic procedure of cardiac catheterization. Young children responded best to nursery rhymes, *Peter and the Wolf,* or *Sesame Street* songs. Older children and teenagers were calmer with rock music, while adults had other favorites.

However, biokinesiologists have found that loud rock music can be weakening, and I do not suggest it for the operating room. Music should serve to calm both the patient and the staff, helping them deal with stress. In the operating room, it should focus everyone's attention on the fact that there is a living person being operated on. It should help the staff relate to that person as though he were awake, rather than distracting them from the surgery. I find that spiritual music and the baroque largo movements recommended in *Superlearning*, by Sheila Ostrander and Lynn Schroeder, are most effective for these purposes. I encourage patients to use tapes of whatever music they find most relaxing or healing, in order to adapt the hospital environment to a healing environment. I also refer you to *The Healing Energies of Music*, by Hal Lingerman, for specific needs. Daniel Kobialka's versions of classical pieces are excellent too.

I've learned what kinds of music are appropriate, and I vary the type according to the surgical situation. I often tease the students by telling them I have specific music to stop bleeding. Sometimes the patient's response leads to an unexpected note of humor. I enjoy spiritual music, and one afternoon, while I was working on a man under spinal anesthesia, the tape came to "Amazing Grace." The patient's head popped up, and he asked, "Is anything wrong down there?" We all laughed and said no. He said, "Well, I'm Irish, and if you'll sing 'When Irish Eyes are Smiling,' I'll feel better." We did, and he enjoyed the performance. One patient, listening to harp music just before the operation began, said, "It's a good thing I heard that while I'm awake. If I woke up and heard it, I wouldn't know where I was." Another day a patient under local anesthesia started laughing and said, "Most appropriate," while I was removing a large benign tumor. In the background Frank Sinatra was singing "Why Not Take All of Me."

DUAL CONTROL

Participation in the decision-making process, more than any other factor, determines the quality of the doctor-patient relationship. The exceptional patient wants to share responsibility for life and treatment, and doctors who encourage that attitude can help all their patients heal faster.

The value of participation has been borne out in two recent studies of children. At the University of Wisconsin Medical School Dr. Charlene Kavanagh compared a group of severely burned children who received standard nursing care with another group who were taught to change their own dressings. Those who had an active role needed less medication and had fewer complications. In Palo Alto, California, a group of asthmatic children were taught about their disease and the drugs used to control it, and encouraged to decide for themselves when they needed medication. They missed far fewer school days and their average rate of emergency-room visits dropped from one a month to one every six months.

Furthermore, shared responsibility increases cooperation and reduces the resentments that often lead to malpractice suits. Second-guessing and recrimination are unlikely when decisions are based on a mutual assessment of what is right for the patient now, not on predictions about the unknowable future. I don't want any of my patients going under anesthesia without feeling that I am doing for them what they wanted done. (However, when certain patients seem likely to be angry at themselves if something goes wrong in the future, based upon their decision, I may suggest they give me more control. I would rather have them mad at me than at themselves. I've done my best, so I can handle their anger.)

Sometimes, when people are subconsciously not sure they want to live, they shy away from the most effective treatment or have so many side effects that it must be stopped. Even when they desperately want to live, they may still disagree with the doctor, who must then fight the impulse to withdraw or coerce. A physician who tries to guarantee the future often pressures the patient into a particular course of treatment, setting them both up for recriminations and feelings of failure if the disease is not cured.

On the other hand, when a patient chooses a form of therapy out of conviction, while accepting the fact that death is inevitable someday, that patient will never be a failure and never regret the decision. The physician must remember that it's the patient who must make the choice and then *live with it.*

It's the physician's duty to accept all patients—though not necessarily to support all their choices. A physician has a right to say, "I can't agree with what you're doing and don't want to participate in it." The sad part is that that kills a lot of people, because they then never go back to a physician. I generally tell such patients, "I don't agree with what you're doing, or if I had your illness I wouldn't choose your plan of treatment, because I don't think you have the best chance of being successful with it, but I will continue to keep a relationship with you, if you wish, and help in any way I can."

Then, if they find that their choice is not productive, they will say, "I know you care about me, because you've kept up the relationship. Will you go ahead and operate on me?" There's no other way a doctor can maximize hope while leaving open a way for the patient later to adopt the treatment recommended by the doctor. Up to this point one hundred percent of my patients have accepted chemotherapy, radiation, or surgery when I have accepted them, even those who initially attempted self-healing and rejected the medical profession. Even those whose initial office visit began with "never talk to me like a doctor! If you do I won't come back."

Acceptance by the physician can help a patient achieve healing and peace, as shown in the case of Bridget, an English woman who had recently moved to New Jersey. Under the English medical system, she'd been assigned a physician, and she didn't like him so she never went back. She had a tumor the size of a melon taking the place of her left breast. I examined her and listed the things I thought could help her, from surgery to God. She said, "You're the first doctor who hasn't screamed and yelled at me, and said, 'Where have you been? Why didn't you come sooner? Why have you been so stupid? What is wrong with you?'" I told her that's not my role. My job is simply to accept patients and try to help them.

I had Bridget draw pictures, which showed unconscious positive attitudes toward radiation and chemotherapy, although consciously she resisted both at first. Several months later she called to tell me that she had started chemotherapy and the tumor had *melted away.* Her response was so dramatic that her oncologist didn't even think she would need radiation. My acceptance of Bridget's condition had enabled her to accept what the medical profession had to offer.

Some surgeons insist on running the whole show, however. They even prohibit their patients from using Reach to Recovery (a post-op emotional and physical therapy program) after mastectomy. They have no right to do so, but some physicians try to take charge of a patient's life as well as the technical details of treatment, like a grownup dominating a child—and the sad truth is that many patients let them. Physicians are created as much by their patients as by their training, and most patients want to give up all decisions to the omnipotent father figure. The exceptional patient fights for responsibility but is punished for this act of survival because he represents a minority of the patients seen by the doctor. As Kostoglotov, the former concentration camp inmate in Aleksandr Solzhenitsyn's *Cancer Ward,* complained to his physician:

No sooner does a patient come to you than you begin to do all his thinking for him. After that, the thinking's done by your standing orders, your five-minute conferences, your program, your plan and the honor of your medical department. And once again I become a grain of sand, just as I was in the camp. Once again nothing *depends* on me.

Critics of modern medicine like to point out the numerous times the death rate has plummeted during doctors' strikes—1976 in Los Angeles, the same year in Bogotá, and 1973 in Jerusalem, for example. They usually say something simplistic, like "Medical care is hazardous to your health." More likely, patients suddenly realize that they have to start looking out for themselves, make their own decisions, as they should have been doing all along, and *that* is what keeps them alive longer. Several years ago there was a strike of ambulance drivers on Cape Cod, where we have a summer house. Panic ensued—what to do with emergencies? Well, the number of emergencies dropped precipitously until the strike was over—another wonderful example of how much control we have.

THE MECHANIC AND THE HEALER

The all too common failure to interact fruitfully with patients comes from the way a physician is taught to be a mere mechanic. In medical school we learn all about disease, but we learn nothing about what disease *means* to the person who has it.

In a study of folk medicine in Taiwan and among Chinese-Americans, Dr. Arthur Kleinman, of the University of Washington School of Medicine, attributed the folk doctor's often surprising success to treatment of sickness in the context of the patient's psychology and culture. The strong stigma attached to mental illness in Chinese society means that a Chinese person often can only conceive of depression, for example, in terms of its physical symptoms, such as fatigue. Hence any treatment that does not allow the patient to believe in a physical cause of the problem is likely to be resisted and remain ineffective.

Kleinman points out a difference between *disease*, defined as the physical or psychiatric symptoms or damage visible to a doctor, and *illness*, the patient's subjective experience of the same sickness. The two are often remarkably different, especially when a person without scientific knowledge is treated by a Western physician.

I don't recommend going into trances or burning spirit money (unless the patient believes only in such methods), but we must, like Plato's free physicians, ask patients what *they* think caused the problem, what threats and losses (or gains) it represents to *them*, and how *they* believe it should be treated. The typical review of systems that medical students are trained to use when questioning patients does not uncover time sequences or the meanings that events have to patients. Even questions like "What did your father die of?" are rarely pursued to find out whether the patient's father died last week or twenty years ago. Therefore, doctors often have no idea of the dynamics of the situation, unless patients volunteer those aspects, which they often don't do.

The best results proceed from a "negotiation" in which the practitioner's viewpoint and that of the patient come close enough together for true communication. If a person fervently believes in religious healing through the laying on of hands, the clinician must not become an obstacle and detract from that treatment's effectiveness. Even if the physician thinks such methods are useless, they are likely to help if the patient believes in them.

I often tell patients how I would treat myself if I had their illness. My choices may not include some of the things they're doing. Likewise, their choices may not include some of the things I would do. But I do not take away the benefit of their methods by saying they're no good. Instead I work to see how our beliefs can mesh. To me the true measure of wholistic medicine is how well the patient and doctor accept each other's belief system, even though their beliefs may differ. Neither one of us forces something upon the other. That way I can say, "If sometimes your beliefs don't work, try mine."

I recently talked to Vivian, a Christian Scientist who said she had been attempting—in vain—to cure herself of a severe bladder infection through prayer. Finally she couldn't stand the pain anymore, so she went to the emergency room. She said a young, inexperienced doctor gave her medication that completely cleared up her symptoms within twenty-four hours. The episode changed her, making her feel that medicines also come from God and should be used along with our inner healing skills.

Obviously, I will try to talk patients out of spending enormous amounts of time and money on something I feel is ineffective, but where positive beliefs are involved I will try to support them. Doing what restores hope is beneficial. Studies show that spending money and traveling a long distance actually help a patient get well. There's a strong urge to be able to say, "I got my money's worth." Moreover, the effort shows a high level of motivation. Such a patient will invariably listen to the physician's advice and act on it. I used to tell patients to mail drawings and call me until I realized the importance of their desire to come. A gentleman from Montana, with cancer of the pancreas, came to me with a 3-month prognosis for survival. He was alive 18 months later because of his hope. Similarly, a willingness to give a little will help the patient accept the doctor's beliefs, allowing the medical therapy a real chance to work. When patients have no faith in the physician's system, they will resist treatment consciously, by not taking their medicine, or unconsciously. In either case, healing will be thwarted.

The value of identifying with the patient explains why the best doctors are often those who've been seriously ill themselves. Throughout our training we learn *not* to empathize with the sick, supposedly to save us psychic strain. All our terminology emphasizes the separation. Instead of a "heart attack," the hospital page operator says "Code 5." The emotional distance hurts both parties, however. We withdraw just when patients need us most. Nurses know how hard it is to find the doctor when a patient is dying. All our education encourages us to think of ourselves as gods of repair, miracle workers. When we can't fix what's broken, we crawl off to lick our wounds, feeling like failures.

The distance also encourages doctors to feel invulnerable: "It's always other people who are sick, not me." When I tell a roomful of medical students, "Almost everybody dies," they all laugh; but when I say the same line to a roomful of doctors, there's dead silence. We become the best deniers of all. As Dr. Gordon Deckert, chief of psychiatry at the University of Oklahoma Medical Center, has observed, "Physicians usually know exactly what they think and believe, but rarely are they in touch with how they feel."

A panel set up by the Association of American Medical Colleges recently concluded that technological specialization is driving out the "exquisite regard for human needs" essential to a doctor's prime goal, the relief of suffering. The main task facing medical schools, said panel chairman Dr. Steven Muller, is to find ways of fostering that regard, which must be taught largely by example.

Instead, the unspoken ideal instilled in college is a medical machismo—the superhumanly tough doc who can handle anything without letting it show. It's okay to be scared of an exam, but admitting a fear of illness and death becomes a sign of weakness.

Naturally, after graduation, we M.D.s deny our sadness at a patient's misfortune, our anger at a patient's resistance, even our joy at a patient's recovery. We are generally very conscientious about our work, but are often unable to relax, play, and recuperate. As a result, we overlook all sorts of warning signals about our own health. No wonder our rates of suicide, drug addiction, and middle-age death are way above average. Just give one of us an airplane and pilot's license, and then ask an actuary what the insurance risk is. "Forget that thunderstorm," the doctor thinks. "I have a meeting to get to. Other people crash, not me."

In a recent article Glen Gabbard, MD, of the Menninger Clinic discussed the role of compulsiveness in the physician creating doubt, guilt, and an exaggerated sense of responsibility. This is reflected in difficulty relaxing, vacationing, and finding family time. In feeling responsible for things beyond one's control, feeling that one is not doing enough, and confusing selfishness and healthy self-interest.

To paraphrase a story of Larry LeShan's: Doctors are busy playing God when so few of us have the qualifications. And besides the job is taken. Playing God leads to self-destruction.

Many colleges are now trying to teach compassion through courses in humanistic medicine, but perhaps the admission of more women to the profession will gradually do more to end this pathetic bravado. The best physicians are those who can find both the "masculine" and "feminine" virtues that exist within their personalities—the ability to make tough decisions and yet remain compassionate and caring. Neither extreme makes a good physician. You can become too involved to make good decisions, and you can also make decisions based on diseases and think nothing of the patient. Combining both is the best way. This has been borne out by studies showing that those who combine both aspects become more effective doctors and also remain happier amid the stresses of their profession.

It's important for most patients to know that their doctors themselves take the advice they give. Yet, feeling immortal, many physicians smoke, drink too much, eat badly and too much, and exercise not at all.

This is sad enough for the physician, but for the patient it's far worse. A sense of invulnerability makes a doctor discount the fears of the patient, who lives in no such charmed fantasy. When someone asks, "What should I eat?" the invincible deity says, "Eat whatever you want. I'm going home and having hot dogs." Asked about the carcinogenic nitrites in them, the physician, behind that invisible shield, laughs.

With such an outlook, we M.D.s sometimes fail to think of the most obvious things, as our son Keith taught me when he was four years old and had to go into the hospital for a hernia repair. I explained all the mechanical details, but when he woke up he said, "You forgot to tell me it was going to hurt." Recently, as a teenager, when he came home with problems, his father had solutions like love-accept-forgive, but he said, "I don't need answers. I need someone to listen." When we play the role of a saint with one-word answers, we don't help people. We help when we listen and share our pain. We must live the sermon, not just deliver it.

A severe staph infection, which once kept me in a hospital for a week, was a crucial part of my education. I found out the difficulties of being in isolation, hooked up to an intravenous line, required to call for help for everything I needed, when I was used to being responsible and in control. I found how hard it is to maintain your dignity in the skimpy gowns that the hospital provides.

This illness came at a time of many changes in my life—a new home, more children, starting practice—all positive events, and yet I became ill. It made me aware that patients in my office must be experiencing similar things. I began to joke with them about changes in *their* lives. I would ask, "Did you get a new job? Did you move to a new house?" They were astonished. How did I know?

I learned more about what doctors were like, too. Since I was a physician, I had eminent professors caring for me, but I couldn't get them all together at one time to give me a straight answer. They even wanted to move me to a more depressing, windowless ward because it was closer to one professor's office. I said no and told them I was leaving the hospital. Suddenly everyone showed up.

I think a few days as a patient on a busy ward should be an integral part of every physician's training—including, as one patient recently added, "an IV in his arm and a tube up his nose." Most tribal cultures recognize a similar necessity. Usually one cannot become a healer without first passing through sickness to health. In our culture, one cannot become a psychoanalyst without being analyzed, but one can become a medical mechanic without ever experiencing the need for repair.

The denial of empathy benefits no one. As mechanics, we doctors always fail in the long run, but as counselors, teachers, healers, and care givers we can always contribute, and even help at the moment of death. Then there's no need to hide in the cafeteria with the beeper and force the nurse to face the patient's death alone. A cooperative arrangement, in which the doctor and patient both realize that they are essentially the same except for a few years' training, offers more to both than the accustomed roles of master and supplicant. In the words of Dr. Francis Peabody, a pioneering medical researcher at Harvard in the 1920s, "The treatment of a disease may be entirely impersonal; the care of a patient must be completely personal . . . the secret of the care of the patient is in caring for the patient."

For most doctors, like myself, the change is long and difficult, but there is no effective alternative. The mental components of all disease make it imperative that the physician be as enlightened, and as much at peace with the self, as a good psychotherapist. In *Modern Man in Search of a Soul,* Carl Jung stated the requirement thus:

And in dealing with himself the doctor must display as much relentlessness, consistency and perseverance as in dealing with his patients. To work upon himself with an equal concentration is truly no small achievement; for he brings to bear all the attentiveness and critical judgment he can summon in showing his patients their mistaken paths, their false conclusions and infantile subterfuges. No one pays the doctor for his introspective efforts; and moreover, we are generally not interested enough in ourselves. Again, we so commonly undervalue the deeper aspects of the human psyche that we hold self-examination or preoccupation with ourselves to be almost morbid. We evidently suspect ourselves of harbouring rather unwholesome things all too reminiscent of a sick-room. The physician must overcome these resistances in himself, for who can educate others while himself uneducated? Who can enlighten his fellows while still in the dark about himself, and who can purify if he is himself unclean? . . . The physician may no longer slip out of his own difficulties by treating the difficulties of others. He will remember that a man who suffers from a running abscess is not fit to perform a surgical operation.

Jung also addressed the need to go beyond a narrow, specialized approach. In his autobiography, *Memories, Dreams, Reflections,* he wrote that, just as physicians learned to use x-rays with no thought of lecturing on subatomic physics, he was "not concerned with proving anything to other disciplines; I am merely attempting to put their knowledge to good use in my own field." Jung broadened psychology by incorporating the perspectives of mythology and philosophy, and, in like manner, today's physicians must apply the insights of psychology and religion to medicine. Later in the same book Jung describes the advantage a doctor derives from this willingness to learn from other fields:

> The difference between most people and myself is that for me the "dividing walls" are transparent. That is my peculiarity. Others find these walls so opaque that they see nothing behind them and therefore think nothing is there. To some extent I perceive the processes going on in the background, and that gives me an inner certainty.

This expanded outlook helps a doctor to inspire hope, give with the heart as well as the head and hands, keep ego in the background, and share major decisions with the patient. Such an approach rewards the physician as well as the patient. The love returns in words and looks of gratitude, in cards and letters, and in little gifts for the office, all of which restore you. A doctor who acts out of love doesn't burn out. He or she may get tired physically, but not emotionally.

The wonders produced by close doctor-patient collaboration never cease to amaze me. One experience illustrates how acceptance can lead a patient to utilize the doctor's recommendations, and also how it can reduce pain. Thelma, a patient with recurrent breast cancer, came to me and said that she wanted God to heal her while I observed and monitored the process. I explained how difficult I thought that would be. On her next visit, the cancer was smaller, and I asked her what had happened. She said, "I left the house with the phone ringing." It was the first time she'd ever said no to anything. Next time, her cancer was even smaller. Again I asked what happened. All smiles, she said, "When my alcoholic husband acted up I called the police. He said, 'You're embarrassing me in front of the neighbors.' I told him, 'I have cancer now, and I don't accept your behavior anymore.' " By the third visit, however, she realized how much I cared for her and we became a team. She said, "It's hard work becoming a saint and healing yourself. Why don't you operate and remove the tumor? I'll work on staying well."

Thelma told me that the night after surgery the nurse came in, pulled the curtain, and said, "Tell me about Dr. Siegel."

My patient responded, "What do you mean? You act like you think he hypnotized me."

The nurse said, "Well, you've had a radical mastectomy, and yet you're walking around the ward cheering up the rest of us, and you have no pain. What did he do to you?"

"He shared with me. This was *our* decision, so there's no reason for me to be depressed or in pain. I know the right thing was done to me by the right person. This is my way of getting well."

Another woman with breast cancer, a young law student named Julie, had terrible fears and dreams about dying under anesthesia. She asked me if I could do the operation under local. I told her, "*I* had a dream in which I did it under local and permanently injured your arm." It was her dream against mine! Our laughter broke the tension. She was able to see my concerns, and, after talking it over some more, she had her mastectomy under general anesthesia with no complications.

Let me explain that this was a fear dream, not a precognitive one. Otherwise I would never have defused it with a joke. If a patient had a dream that I felt predicted that person's death, I would not operate that day. For example, one patient dreamed of her headstone with "Thursday" engraved on it, so we made sure her surgery was not done on a Thursday.

The day after Julie's operation I was at a seminar in a

nearby town. A familiar voice asked a question from the audience. It was Julie. I rushed over to ask what in the world she was doing there. She said, "Don't worry. All the tubes are under my dress. When I had no pain and wanted to leave, the nurses said, 'Oh, she's just another one of Dr. Siegel's patients,' and your partner signed the discharge order."

It isn't me, though. It's the relationship that makes such results possible. It's sharing and caring, doing things *for* people, not *to* them. We physicians must become instruments. When that happens, motivated patients will use us to work miracles. Just how fundamentally we can change the patient's reaction to our treatments has been exquisitely captured by Page Coulter, one of my patients, in her poem "Repairs." Even the title points up the difference between a cooperative approach and the typical medical talk of "assaulting," "mutilating," or "insulting" the body in order to heal it. After showing how her fears were calmed by a gentle anesthesiologist, she continues:

> We could justify the need for love, or crack open
> the eye of a tulip.
> Who cares? We try to stretch our bodies to catch the
> rain
> Or fallout or darkness, anything that falls from
> outer space.
> But instead I hear the surgeon singing "Desert
> Song,"
> And I feel his gentle tugs and pulls as though it
> were my father
> Caning chairs or my mother sewing pockets in my
> wedding dress.

3

*The great majority of us are required to live a life of
constant, systematic duplicity. Your health is bound to
be affected if, day after day, you say the opposite of
what you feel, if you grovel before what you dislike
and rejoice at what brings you nothing but misfortune.
Our nervous system isn't just a fiction, it's a part of our
physical body, and our soul exists in space and is
inside us, like the teeth in our mouth. It can't be
forever violated with impunity.*

—BORIS PASTERNAK, *Doctor Zhivago*

Disease and the Mind

Neglect of the mind-body link by technological medicine is
actually a brief aberration when viewed against the whole
history of the healing art. In traditional tribal medicine and in
Western practice from its beginning in the work of Hippocrates, the need to operate through the patient's mind has always been recognized. Until the nineteenth century, medical
writers rarely failed to note the influence of grief, despair, or
discouragement on the onset and outcome of illness, nor did
they ignore the healing effects of faith, confidence, and peace
of mind. Contentment used to be considered a prerequisite for
health.

The modern medicine man has gained so much power
over certain diseases through drugs, however, that he has forgotten about the potential strength within the patient. One
elderly physician friend recently told me of reading the diary
of his uncle, also a doctor. In the early years, the diarist always
recorded what happened to the individual or the community
prior to an illness or epidemic, but as medicine became more
technological, this part of the history grew less and less important to him and finally was omitted altogether. Awareness of
the mind's powers was lost as medicine cast out all "soft" data,
the information that's not easily quantified or scientific.

THE MIND—BENIGN OR MALIGN

Part of the mind's effect on health is direct and conscious. The extent to which we love ourselves determines whether we eat right, get enough sleep, smoke, wear seat belts, exercise, and so on. Each of these choices is a statement of how much we care about living. These decisions control about 90 percent of the factors that determine our state of health. The trouble is that most people's motivation to attend to these basics is deflected by attitudes hidden from everyday awareness. As a result, many of us have mixed intentions.

Consider, for example, Sara, a woman who came to me with breast cancer a few years ago; she was smoking when I walked into her hospital room. Her action clearly stated: "I want you to get rid of my cancer, but I'm ambivalent about living, so I think I'll risk a second cancer." She looked up sheepishly and said, "I suppose you're going to tell me to stop smoking."

"No," I said, "I'm going to tell you to love yourself. Then you'll stop."

She thought for a moment and replied, "Well, I do love myself. I just don't adore myself." (Sara ultimately did come to adore herself—and stopped smoking.)

It was a good quip, but it exemplified an important problem many people have with themselves. Self-love has come to mean only vanity and narcissism. The pride of being and the determination to care for our own needs have gone out of the meaning. Nevertheless, an unreserved, positive self-adoration remains the essence of health, the most important asset a patient must gain to become exceptional. Self-esteem and self-love are not sinful. They make living a joy instead of a chore.

The mind does not act only through our conscious choices, however. Many of its effects are achieved directly on the body's tissues, without any awareness on our part. Consider some of our common expressions: "He's a pain in the neck/ass. Get off my back. This problem is eating me up alive. You're breaking my heart." The body responds to the mind's messages, whether conscious or unconscious. In general, these may be either "live" or "die" messages. I am convinced we not only have survival mechanisms, such as the fight-or-flight response, but also a "die" mechanism that actively stops our defenses, slowing the body's functions and bringing us toward death when we feel our life is not worth living.

Every tissue and organ in the body is controlled by a complex interaction among chemicals circulating in the bloodstream, the hormones secreted by our endocrine glands. This mixture is controlled by the "master gland," the pituitary gland, located in the middle of the head just below the brain. The output of pituitary hormones in turn is controlled by both chemical secretions and nerve impulses from the neighboring part of the brain, called the hypothalamus. This tiny region regulates most of the body's unconscious maintenance processes, such as heartbeat, breathing, blood pressure, temperature, and so forth.

Nerve fibers enter the hypothalamus from nearly all other regions of the brain, so that intellectual and emotional processes occurring elsewhere in the brain affect the body. For example, about five years ago, child-development researchers discovered "psychosocial dwarfism," a disturbingly common syndrome in which an unhealthy emotional atmosphere at home stunts a child's physical growth. When a child is caught in a crossfire of hostility and feels rejected by his or her parents, thereby growing up with little self-esteem, the brain's emotional center, or limbic system, acts upon the nearby hypothalamus to shut off the pituitary gland's production of growth hormone.

The immune system consists of more than a dozen different types of white blood cells concentrated in the spleen, thymus gland, and lymph nodes, and patrolling the entire body through the blood and lymphatic systems. They are divided into two main types. One group, called B cells, produce chemicals that neutralize poisons made by disease organisms while helping the body mobilize its own defenses. The other group, called T cells, consists of killer cells and their helpers, which destroy invading bacteria and viruses.

Recent research has shown heretofore unknown nerves connecting the thymus and spleen directly to the hypothalamus. Other work has proven that white blood cells re-

spond directly to some of the same chemicals that carry messages from one nerve cell to another.

This anatomical evidence for direct control of the immune
system by the brain has been confirmed in studies of animals.
Two groups of scientists have independently used Pavlovian
conditioning techniques to change the immune response. At
the University of Rochester Medical Center, psychiatrist Robert Ader and immunologist Nicholas Cohen repeatedly gave
rats saccharin-sweetened water along with an immune-sup-
pressant drug. Later they were able to "trick" the animals into
suppressing their own immune responses by giving them the
sweetened water alone. Working for the National Institutes of
Health, Dr. Novera Herbert Spector similarly conditioned
mice to *increase* their immune responses when exposed to the
smell of camphor.

The immune system, then, is controlled by the brain, either indirectly through hormones in the bloodstream, or directly through the nerves and neurochemicals. One of the
most widely accepted explanations of cancer, the "surveil-
lance" theory, states that cancer cells are developing in our
bodies all the time but are normally destroyed by white blood
cells before they can develop into dangerous tumors. Cancer
appears when the immune system becomes suppressed and
can no longer deal with this routine threat. It follows that
whatever upsets the brain's control of the immune system will
foster malignancy.

This disruption occurs primarily by means of the chronic
stress syndrome first described by Hans Selye in 1936. The
mixture of hormones released by the adrenal glands as part of
the fight-or-flight response suppresses the immune system.
This was all right in dealing with the occasional threats our
ancestors faced from wild beasts. However, when the tension
and anxiety of modern life keep the stress response "on" continually, the hormones lower our resistance to disease, even
withering away the lymph nodes. Moreover, there is now experimental evidence that "passive emotions," such as grief,
feelings of failure, and suppression of anger, produce over-
secretion of these same hormones, which suppress the immune system.

We don't yet understand all the ways in which brain chemicals are related to emotions and thoughts, but the salient point is that our state of mind has an immediate and direct effect on our state of body. We can change the body by dealing with how we feel. If we ignore our despair, the body receives a "die" message. If we deal with our pain and seek help, then the message is "Living is difficult but desirable," and the immune system works to keep us alive.

I therefore use two major tools to change the body—emotions and imagery. These are the two ways we can get our minds and bodies to communicate with each other. Our emotions and words let the body know what we expect of it, and by visualizing certain changes we can help the body bring them about. Both emotions and imagery are obviously transmitted through the central nervous system and may relate to work that Robert Becker, an orthopedic surgeon and researcher, has done.

Becker has studied the body's electrical systems. His work led directly to the use of electricity to heal broken bones that have failed to knit. Becker found that hypnotized patients can produce voltage changes in specific areas of the body on command. If these voltages control the chemical and cellular processes of healing, as Becker believes, then we soon may have a scientific explanation for hypnosis cures and the placebo effect. It is well known, for example, that hypnotized patients can cure their own warts. As Lewis Thomas wrote in *The Medusa and the Snail:*

You can't sit there under hypnosis, taking suggestions in and having them acted on with such accuracy and precision, without assuming the existence of something very like a controller. It wouldn't do to fob off the whole intricate business on lower centers without sending along a quite detailed set of specifications, way over my head.

Some intelligence or other knows how to get rid of warts, and this is a disquieting thought.

It is also a wonderful problem, in need of solving. Just think what we would know, if we had anything like a clear understanding of what goes on when a wart is hypnotized away.

. . . we would be finding out about a kind of superintelligence that exists in each of us, infinitely smarter and possessed of technical know-how far beyond our present understanding. It would be worth a War on Warts, a Conquest of Warts, a National Institute of Warts and all.

Bioelectricity may someday enable us to reach this "controller" directly, to understand exactly how and why tumors sometimes regress when patients are convinced that an unorthodox treatment—hypnosis, diet, prayer, meditation—is going to work. As Becker once wrote to me, "The placebo effect is not only real but of great importance, and your methods may be far more effective than you think they are."

Whether or not we can ever control all healing with electrical stimuli, exceptional patients—that is, potentially *all* patients—need not wait helplessly for artificial aids. They can learn to heal themselves and stay well. If I can teach you how to feel good about your life, love yourself and others, and achieve peace of mind, the necessary changes can occur. My loving and hugging may look silly on the ward, but they're scientific. The problem is that we don't yet know the psychological techniques necessary to turn on the healing process quickly and efficiently in everyone. So many of the changes happen at an unconscious level that they are hard to measure clinically without careful psychological testing. One day I hope we can prescribe something like "one hug every three hours" instead of a drug or electrical impulse, but for the moment we must return to our consideration of the mind's potential for harm, as a prelude to finding its antidote.

COPING WITH STRESS

It's often said that stress is one of the most destructive elements in people's daily lives, but that's only a half truth. The way we react to stress appears to be more important than the stress itself. This was borne out in the experience of Hans Selye, the scientist who developed the entire concept of stress and its effects on the body.

At age sixty-five, Selye developed reticulum cell sarcoma, a type of cancer whose cure rate is extremely low. This is perhaps the ultimate stress, but in an interview Selye discussed how he reacted to it in an exceptional way:

"I was sure I was going to die, so I said to myself, 'All right now, this is about the very worst thing that could happen to you, but there are two ways you can handle this; either you can go around feeling like a miserable candidate on death row and whimper away a year, or else you can try to squeeze as much from life now as you can.' I chose the latter because I'm a fighter, and cancer provided me with the biggest fight of my life. I took it as a natural experiment that pushed me to the ultimate test whether I was right or wrong. Then a strange thing happened. A year went by, then two, then three, and look what happened. It turned out that I was that fortunate exception. . . ."

"Afterward I made a particular effort to cut down my stress level. I have to be very careful what I say here because I am a scientist, and no statistics now exist to say whether stress is related to cancer. Apart from the genetic and environmental causes of cancer, I can only say that the relationship between stress and cancer is rather complicated. In just the same way that electricity can both cause and prevent heat, depending on how things are balanced, stress can both initiate and prevent illness."

[The interviewer asked,] "Some people have described cancer as a disease that is somewhat like the body's way of rejecting itself. Now to carry that premise one step further, could it be that when people drastically reject their basic needs they are possibly more apt to develop cancer? In other words, if a person rejects his own needs, can his body rebel and reject itself?"

[Selye said,] "I don't say yes and I don't say no. I'm a scientist, not a philosopher. All I can say as a scientist is that the great majority of physical illnesses have in part some psychosomatic origin."

The evidence gathered since Dr. Selye wrote these words suggests he was overly cautious. In particular, the onset and course of disease are strongly linked to a person's ability and willingness to cope with stress. Stresses that we *choose* evoke a response totally different from those we'd like to avoid but cannot. Helplessness is worse than the stress itself. This is probably why the rate of cancer is higher for blacks in America than for whites, and why cancer is associated with grief and depression. Those most likely to die of heart attacks are not the hard-driving Type A executives but rather those who are driven, the underlings and factory workers who have no autonomy and whose shortened lives give new meaning to the phrase "deadly boredom."

The interpretation of stress is always tricky for an outsider, for the same circumstances can be detrimental to one and neutral or even beneficial to another. Johns Hopkins University psychiatrist Jerome Frank, citing a 1961 study by L. E. Hinkle, notes that "stress comes mainly from the patient's interpretation of events." In Hinkle's long-term study of the subject, life experiences that seemed benign to an objective observer were often felt as stressful by the patients and associated with illness. Conversely, stresses that appeared horrendous to the observer—such as poverty, bereavement, alcoholism in the family—usually were not associated with illnesses if the patients did not report them as stressful.

This is especially true in the case of children. Adults often assume that children are happy when they are actually being traumatized by events, even though they often don't show it. Children have been known to commit suicide over receiving a B instead of an A on a report card, because they internalized their parents' expectations, or reacted to a comment that made them feel unloved.

But the scientific mind is seldom convinced by psychological studies on humans. There are just too many variables for a researcher to control them all. Tests on animals have yielded conclusive evidence, however. In the mid-1970s the late Vernon Riley, at Seattle's Pacific Northwest Research Foundation, completed a thorough series of experiments with a strain of mice bred to be susceptible to breast cancer. By raising some in sheltered, stress-free environments and others in stressful surroundings, he was able to vary the rate of cancer from 7 to 92 percent.

A 1981 experiment by a team of three psychologists proved the point with an even better simulation of the human experience. Madelon Visintainer and two co-workers injected three groups of rats with live tumor cells. One day later they subjected two of the groups to electric shock. The stress was administered so that one group could not evade it, while the other rats were warned by a signal so they could escape by jumping over a barrier. Of the helpless rats, 73 percent came down with the cancer, while only 37 percent of the other group developed it. They did slightly better than the control group, which received no shocks at all!

The level of stress is determined partly by society. Cultures that place the highest value on a combination of individualism and competition are the most stressful. Those that seem to produce the least stress and have the lowest rates of cancer are close-knit communities in which supportive, loving relationships are the norm, and the elderly retain an active role. Religious faith and a fairly open, accepting attitude toward sexuality are two other common characteristics of low-cancer societies.

These are some of the same circumstances that favor longevity. Soviet Georgia, the Hunza valley, Mormon communities in America, and the villages of the Abujmarhia tribe of central India are excellent examples. The Abujmarhia enjoy a pollution-free environment, a wholesome natural diet, abundantly loving sexual relationships beginning premaritally in early adolescence, relaxed but occasionally strenuous work in the fields by day, dancing and storytelling by evening, and plenty of rest. Cancer is absolutely unknown among them.

It must be noted that these societies don't invest time and effort to help malformed infants survive, so physical factors determined by natural selection also influence disease rates. Still, externals are not the whole story. Environmental purity and death from genetic defects still prevail in other undeveloped areas, but cancer is more common among tribes who regularly engage in warfare than among those who live at peace.

The security of routine also seems to help limit serious disease. Closed structured societies in which all members know what is expected of them, even when deviation from the norm is not tolerated—Mormons, Seventh Day Adventists, and Mennonites in the United States, for example—have lower rates of disease than the surrounding, more open society.

When individuals leave the cluster for a life with more unknowns, their incidence of disease reaches that in the culture they enter.

In a society like ours, the response to stress is left to the individual, who must learn to disconnect psychologically from external pressures. Dr. Herbert Benson of Harvard Medical School has shown that the ability to maintain a healthy cholesterol level is directly related to the ability to handle stress through relaxation. With meditation and exercise, we can teach hard-driving, success-oriented (Type A) persons to avoid heart attacks while keeping their Type A behavior. Studies of people who meditate regularly have shown that their physiological age is much lower than their chronological age. These techniques do people no good without the motivation to use them. The first requirement is to get people to love themselves enough to care for their bodies and minds.

Stress can be measured. One of the yardsticks for it, developed by Drs. Thomas Holmes and Richard Rahe, uses a list of forty-three stressful changes to assess a person's likelihood of becoming ill. The evaluation begins with a history of the persons's recent emotional life, then assigns a certain number of "points" to each life crisis, such as changing or losing a job, children leaving for college, marriage or divorce, moving to a new house, and so on.

The highest value, 100 points, is attached to the most grievous loss, the death of one's spouse. This most traumatic of events is often followed by cancer or other catastrophic illness in one or two years. Recent studies have confirmed that grieving spouses have depressed immune systems for over a year. Additional work has shown that *within one day* any uncontrollable stress lowers the efficiency of the body's disease-fighting killer cells.

New evidence suggests that divorce may be even more devastating to many people, since it's harder to accept that the relationship is really over. Indeed, divorced people have higher rates of cancer, heart disease, pneumonia, high blood pressure, and accidental death than married, single, or widowed persons. Married men also have one-third the lung-cancer incidence of single men and can smoke three times as much with the same cancer incidence as single men.

Career reversals also commonly lead to malignancy. The defeats of Napoleon Bonaparte, Ulysses S. Grant, William Howard Taft, and Hubert Humphrey have often been implicated in their fatal cancers.

One of the arguments of those who discount mental factors in cancer has been the notion that the latency period is too long for the mind to play a role in childhood cancer, but there is now evidence to the contrary. A study at the Albert Einstein College of Medicine in the Bronx found that children with cancer had had twice as many recent crises as other children matched to be similar except for their disease. Another study showed that 31 of 33 children with leukemia had experienced a traumatic loss or move within the two years before their diagnosis. Psychologists are now learning that infants are far more perceptive than heretofore imagined, and I wouldn't be surprised if cancer in early childhood was linked to messages of parental conflict or disapproval perceived even in the womb. I don't say this to create guilt but to give us more insight into our participation in the healing process.

In dealing with the problems presented by cancer, therefore, we must not forget the effects this crisis may have on family and friends, particularly if the patient dies. The doctor must help the others deal with their fears and grief openly, in an effort to prevent further disease. When stress is confronted and love is shared, everyone—the family as well as the patient —benefits.

QUIET DESPERATION

Not everyone who suffers a tragic loss or stressful change in lifestyle develops an illness. The deciding factor seems to be how one copes with the problem. Those who can give vent to their feelings yet continue with their lives generally stay well.

The husband of a patient once called me up and asked, "What did you tell my wife?" He said she came home and yelled at him for hours about their twenty years of marriage

—and he thought they had been pretty good. I told him, "I didn't say anything to your wife, but she has learned that she has cancer, and she's sharing the resentment that she has built up over the years." Anger is a normal emotion if it is expressed when it is felt. If it isn't it develops into resentment or even hatred, which can be very destructive. A woman who says, "I'll make this marriage work if it kills me" may find it will.

If a person deals with anger or despair when they first appear, illness need not occur. When we don't deal with our emotional needs, we set ourselves up for physical illness. Yet what are most of us more comfortable with—telling the neighbors we have to see a psychiatrist or that we need an operation? We're uncomfortable saying we're being driven crazy but not that we're being driven to illness.

The simple truth is, happy people generally don't get sick. One's attitude toward oneself is the single most important factor in healing or staying well. Those who are at peace with themselves and their immediate surroundings have far fewer serious illnesses than those who are not.

In one of the most thorough studies of this "contentment factor," psychiatrist George Vaillant followed two hundred Harvard graduates for thirty years, correlating health surveys with psychological tests each year. Comparing the happiest versus the unhappiest group, he reported: "Of 59 men with the best mental health assessed from the age of 21 to 46 years, only two became chronically ill or died by the age of 53. Of the 48 men with the worst mental health from the age of 21 to 46, 18 became chronically ill or died." Those who were extremely satisfied with their lives had *one-tenth* the rate of serious illness and death suffered by their thoroughly dissatisfied peers. The findings remained valid when the effects of alcohol, tobacco, obesity, and ancestral longevity were statistically eliminated— even though unhappiness obviously can contribute to all but the last variable. Mental health, Vaillant found, retards mid-life deterioration in physical health.

The common denominator in all depression is a lack of love or a loss of meaning in life, at least as perceived from the depressed person's point of view. Illness then often functions as an escape from a routine that has become meaningless. In this sense it might even be called a Western form of meditation.

One of the most common precursors of cancer is a traumatic loss or a feeling of emptiness in one's life. When a salamander loses a limb, it grows a new one. In an analogous way, when a human being suffers an emotional loss that is not properly dealt with, the body often responds by developing a new growth. It appears that if we can react to loss with personal growth, we can prevent growth gone wrong within us. In like manner, researchers have found, if a salamander is given cancer on a limb or tail and the appendage is then amputated near the tumor, a new limb or tail appears and the cancer cells become normal again. We know that the human body tries to heal some cancers, such as neuroblastoma, by changing the malignant cells back to normal in the same way, as well as by attacking them. Thus it is my main job as a doctor to help you develop into a new person so you can resist the unwanted, uncontrolled development of illness.

If I transplant a kidney into you and give you drugs that inhibit your immune system, the graft will take. Later we may find that the transplanted kidney contained a cancer. The kidney and cancer will both thrive. If I take away the drugs that keep your body from rejecting the kidney, the new organ will be destroyed, and so will the cancer. A vigorous immune system can overcome cancer if it is not interfered with, and emotional growth toward greater self-acceptance and fulfillment helps keep the immune system strong.

Depression's effects on the immune system often appear very quickly if some remnant of a previous disease remains. Arnold, a patient who had had malignant melanoma and had been in remission for seven years, came to me with a recurrence in a lymph node in his armpit. I asked what had happened in his life during the last six months. He told me he had brought up all his children himself, because his wife had been mentally ill. The last child, a son to whom he was especially close, had just gotten married and left home. He'd been so depressed by his son's departure that he'd cried for weeks.

Despair had depressed Arnold's immune response, allowing residual cancer cells that had been under control to multiply again. As part of his therapy we brought together his children and the rest of the family, to help plan new interests and social activities for him, as well as to find ways in which the others could remain close to him. He was able to understand the physical danger of sinking into despair and self-pity. He began to participate in staying well by learning to deal with the unavoidable emotional problems of his life. He eventually died of his disease, but his remaining time was filled with happiness from the love of his family, new friends, and a girlfriend.

Depression as defined by psychologists generally involves quitting or giving up. Feeling that present conditions and future possibilities are intolerable, the depressed person "goes on strike" from life, doing less and less, and losing interest in people, work, hobbies, and so on. Such depression is strongly linked with cancer. Dr. Bernard Fox of Boston, for example, found that depressed men are twice as likely to get cancer as nondepressives. A study of identical twins, one of whom in each pair had leukemia, showed that the one with the disease had become severely depressed or suffered an emotional loss beforehand, while the healthy twin had not. However, there is a specific form of depression even more closely related to malignancy.

Typical depressed patients, by abdicating normal activity, are at least offering some response to what they perceive as an unbearable situation. The reaction is negative, but at least it's an attempt to back away. Many people, however, continue with their routines and an outward show of happiness, when on the inside their lives have come to lack all meaning. These persons are seldom diagnosed as clinically depressed, because they manage to keep functioning. Their state is the "quiet desperation" of James Thurber's Walter Mitty, meek and obliging on the outside, but filled with unacknowledged rage and frustration.

A cancer patient named Sandy, for example, wrote me a long letter explaining how she'd become conditioned to be a "doormat" most of her life. In her teens she'd trained as a singer and actress, even studying in a noted experimental theater group. She told me that, each time she came off the stage flushed with excitement, her mother would say, "It was good. Keep practicing and maybe *next time* you'll do better." Her mother likewise greeted every report card with *"Next time* see if you can bring me all A's." Sandy had a lovely, voluptuous figure, but her mother always told her, "Don't eat this, don't eat that, you're too fat." By her late teens, Sandy's self-confidence was so low that she only sang at the back of the church choir, and pretty soon not even there.

Then, just out of high school, Sandy got married:

We never knew each other until it was too late. Being Catholic, I had to try to make it work out. We had three kids, three years apart. . . . [My husband] worked two jobs—I did odd jobs cleaning houses whenever I could. My Mother was there every day "to see the kids," and she would constantly remind me that no one would hire me because I was too fat and that, besides, what could I ever do to earn any money? When I reminded her that I used to be a legal secretary . . . she would brush that off with, "Well, you can't go to work until the kids are in school. I can't take care of them, they are too much work, and I forbid you to have strangers raising my grandchildren."

Sandy was always getting sick, and her mother was always there reminding her how tired she must be and how ungrateful she was for all her mother did for her. Her husband started staying out all night, then coming home drunk and beating her up. When she asked him for a divorce, he put the whole family in the car, took them to the edge of a cliff and threatened to drive off unless she promised never again to talk of leaving him. She made the promise and kept it.

Although she tried to keep up appearances, Sandy decided, on an unconscious level, to be sick. She developed phlebitis and stayed in bed all the time, having no relationship with her husband. After he was killed in an auto accident, her phlebitis cleared up within days. Later, during a second marriage in which she again took a subordinate role, Sandy developed breast cancer. At that time she redirected her life and is well today.

During more than two decades of research into the mental aspects of cancer, experimental psychologist Lawrence LeShan conducted personality studies of 455 cancer patients and in-depth therapy of 71 "terminal" cases. He found that this condition of "despair" (so named to distinguish it from the more commonly recognized form of depression) was reported as predating the disease by 68 of his 71 cancer patients in therapy, but by only 3 of 88 other clients who did not have cancer. In *The Will to Live* Arnold Hutschnecker wrote, "Depression is a partial surrender to death, and it seems that cancer is despair experienced at the cellular level."

The relationship between cancer and withheld emotion was put on a scientific basis over thirty years ago when internist D. M. Kissen studied a group of smokers, comparing those who had lung cancer with those having other diseases. Based on personality tests, Kissen found the cancer patients had poorer "outlets for emotional discharge," and concluded that, the more repressed a person was, the fewer cigarettes were needed to cause cancer.

Working with breast-cancer patients, Mogens Jensen of the Yale psychology department showed that "defensive-repressors" die faster than patients with a more realistic outlook. These are the smiling ones who don't acknowledge their desperation, who say, "I'm fine," even though you know they have cancer, their spouses have run off, their children are drug addicts, and the house just burned down. Jensen feels this behavior "disregulates" and exhausts the immune system because it is confused by the mixed messages.

Thus, when a patient tells me he or she is fine, I have to know whether it's a performance or the truth. One must be careful when evaluating a patient who says cancer is not stressful. It may not be if it's a solution to life's problems. Then again, if one can face the disease with peace of mind instead of fear, it becomes a challenging stress rather than a purely destructive one. The outcomes will be different, and they will not be interpreted properly unless the attitudes are carefully measured by psychological testing.

Jensen also noted that those with imagery or daydreams that were always positive, in the sense of denying illness or the possibility of death, had a poor chance of survival. Imaging techniques don't work with people who deny, because they can't accept their illness and therefore don't really participate in fighting it. In drawings, defensive-repressors depict themselves with enormous smiles, portraying the illness outside their bodies on another page, or representing their own bodies with pictures of healthy bodies cut out of magazines. One such woman told me, "I'm not a good artist, so I had my ten-year-old son draw a picture." (Later, after I asked how she expected to get over cancer if she didn't even have the courage to do a picture, she did draw her own.)

Psychiatrist George Engel surveyed the evidence and concluded that the most important factor in bringing on despair is usually a change in the environment about which the patient feels powerless—in other words, he or she has a sense of hopelessness and helplessness. Sudden death often follows these changes. Such deaths sometimes occur with amazing speed, as when a spouse of fifty years dies and the survivor collapses and dies ten minutes later.

Both men and women are subject to hopelessness, but because of their often divergent roles, the situations that trigger it are often different. Men typically get sick soon after losing a job or retiring, because they have traditionally identified more strongly with their work than women have. My own father developed lung cancer shortly after retiring. At first it was hard for him to admit the significance of his retirement. Fortunately, after surgery, he was able to find fulfillment in his life, and the disease has not recurred in over twelve years.

Men are generally better able to express anger, while women tend to hold it in and become depressed. For them the change generally happens in the home. It may be a divorce or the growing up and departure of children. As a woman who developed cancer after her children left home expressed it in a letter to me, "I had an empty place in me, and cancer grew to fill it."

The cause may simply be a gradual dissatisfaction with the role of housewife, if that role is unfulfilling for the woman. It is not the role itself, but rather the feeling of being trapped.

Housewives get 54 percent more cancer than the general population, and 157 percent more than women who work outside the home. When these results were first published, by Dr. William Morton of the University of Oregon, many researchers assumed there must be a carcinogen in the kitchen, and much fruitless research was spent looking for it. Now, there may well be some carcinogens in many American kitchens, but a further statistical analysis revealed that salaried domestics have *less* cancer than housewives, despite working in *two* kitchens. However, most research funds still are allocated to look for chemical causes. Little thought has been given to the possibility that the housewife's high risk of cancer may be due to her feeling trapped and the fact that often she is not living the life she wants but a performance.

In a ballad called "Miss Gee," W. H. Auden poignantly expressed the relationship between disease and a loveless, frustrated life:

> She bicycled down to the doctor,
>   And rang the surgery bell;
> "O, doctor, I've a pain inside me,
>   And I don't feel very well."
>
> Doctor Thomas looked her over,
>   And then he looked some more;
> Walked over to his wash-basin,
>   Said, "Why didn't you come before?"
>
> Doctor Thomas sat over his dinner.
>   Though his wife was waiting to ring;*
> Rolling his bread into pellets;
>   Said, "Cancer's a funny thing.
>
> "Nobody knows what the cause is,
>   Though some pretend they do;
> It's like some hidden assassin
>   Waiting to strike at you.

*For a servant to clear the table.

"Childless women get it,
And men when they retire;
It's as if there had to be some outlet
For their foiled creative fire."

A psychiatrist once told me, "Not everything that rhymes is true," but I rather subscribe to Lawrence LeShan's outlook. Before he begins new research, he reads to see whether poets and artists have already expressed the same ideas. If they have, he proceeds, knowing he's on the right track.

Lack of emotional outlet is a common theme in the histories of cancer patients. It is probably the reason cancer is more common in convents than in prisons: in jail you can at least act out your frustrations. One of LeShan's patients was a former gang leader who developed Hodgkin's disease when his exciting life—surrounded by supporters and danger—ended. The gang grew up and disbanded. The young man felt bored with his life and showed no response to therapy. As the issues became clear, LeShan encouraged him to join the fire department, which brought male camaraderie and danger back into his life. Soon his body began to respond, and the disease receded. A new problem appeared when he was offered a promotion. His wife wanted him to accept, but he was afraid taking a desk job would imperil his recovery. Time will tell whether he has grown enough to choose the right course.

To some extent, then, cancer is not a primary disease. It is partly a reaction to a set of circumstances that weaken the body's defenses. That is why, when a doctor cures cancer or some other disease without ensuring that the treatment addresses the patient's entire life, a new illness may appear. Since everyone is subject to external changes, truly effective treatment must get a patient to become the kind of person who can live comfortably and happily in spite of such stresses. This process is never complete, but it is the process itself that benefits our bodies. One does not have to *be* a saint to be healed. It's the effort of working *toward* sainthood that brings the rewards. As Richard Bach, author of *Jonathan Livingston Sea-*

gull, wrote, "Here's a test to find whether your mission on earth is finished: If you're alive, it isn't."

PERSONALITY PROGRAMMING

As a young woman, my mother had severe hyperthyroidism and weighed about ninety pounds. She also desperately wanted a child. She went to many obstetricians, but they all said her body couldn't stand the strain and she would probably die if she became pregnant. After several years during which her condition didn't improve, she and my father decided a baby was worth the risk. At that point she became an exceptional patient: she began to share her hopes and fears with her doctors, dealing with them on the emotional as well as the intellectual level, and my mother and father took ultimate responsibility for the decision to have a child.

Finally my parents found one obstetrician who was willing to help my mother take the chance. He told her he would support her in her attempt to carry through a normal pregnancy if she could gain thirty pounds. My mother had a wonderful asset at home—a Jewish mother. She took her daughter home, had her lie down on the couch, and fed her constantly for three months. My mother gained the required weight and conceived, and I was born. Her hyperthyroidism disappeared after my birth, and my parents had the gift of a healthy infant.

The delivery was traumatic. At first my features were grossly distorted from the forceps. When my mother took me for walks in the carriage, she covered it to hide me. Neighbors would stop, lift the cover, and start to coo, "Oh, what a cute . . ." until they caught a glimpse, saw that the usual phrases weren't appropriate, and were left gaping. My mother decided to keep me home and save the neighbors embarrassment. There are no baby pictures from these early months, which proves it. My grandmother stepped in, anointing and stroking my face until the damage healed, relieving my mother of her distress and continuing the unconditional love.

So I received the message that I was loved unconditionally, even more strongly than babies who enter life under easier circumstances. I know that I have my parents' support and love no matter what I choose to do. I am absolutely convinced that the feeling of support I grew up with gave me the belief that I could be what I wanted to be and guided me toward my desire to give and to heal.

These first experiences conditioned me to be a survivor. Life became a series of obstacles that I always felt I could overcome. If I was not valued by others, I knew I could count on my family and the self-esteem they helped me develop. In a sense, this was a handicap for me as a physician, because I didn't realize what went on in other people's lives.

The hardest lesson for me to learn was that most of my patients are not the products of such love. In fact, I would estimate that 80 percent of my patients were unwanted or treated indifferently as children. Even laboratory rats, when prematurely separated from their mothers, become more susceptible to cancer. Rats that are frequently petted in infancy become less susceptible. How dissimilar my experience from those who hear "We always wanted a boy instead of a girl," or "Your father was drunk—we didn't want more children," or even "I wish I'd had an abortion instead of you." Such messages lead to a lifelong feeling of unworthiness. Then an illness is something the patient deserves, and treatment becomes undeserved. For such people the disease can be their way of finally satisfying their parents' wishes—or God's, since many people carry a burden of guilt from their religion, experiencing illness as punishment for sin. At bottom, they feel that the only way they can be really good or receive love is by dying.

One of my patients was a New Yorker named Jan, who'd been an actress since her early teens. Her mother had constantly warned her to protect her breasts, since they were all-important for her appearance. She told her she shouldn't sleep on her stomach, and when she danced she should be careful no one bumped them. Naturally, Jan got breast cancer and couldn't consider surgery. Instead she tried every alternative therapy on the market. I told her that if she could concentrate her incredible energy on one or two choices and learn to love herself, she would have a great chance for a cure. But, like many performers, she lived mainly for the approval of others.

She said, "If I don't hear any applause, how do I know I'm lovable?" She died of her disease, burning away her energy looking for an outside miracle.

The miracles come from within. *You are not that unloved child anymore.* You *can* be reborn, rejecting the old messages and their consequent diseases. When you choose to love you will have those days when you're not all you'd like to be, but you *can* learn to forgive yourself. You can't change your short-comings until you accept yourself despite them. I emphasize this because many people, especially those at high risk of can-cer, are prone to forgive others and crucify themselves. I see all of us as being perfectly imperfect, and ask that we accept ourselves that way. As Elisabeth Kübler-Ross says, "I'm not okay, you're not okay, but that's okay."

The remaining chapters will show how personality repro-gramming is done, but let me give you a little example here from my own experience. The problem—seasickness—is un-doubtedly trivial compared with cancer, but the principles are the same, and the episode taught me how powerful and poten-tially dangerous the mind is.

One summer I was reading a book whose authors recom-mended as a technique for losing weight that you visualize yourself feeling sick as you approached the dinner table. I was enthusiastic about trying all these exercises, and I had also gotten dreadfully seasick since childhood every time I'd gone out on choppy water. In fact, I'd recently gone fishing on vacation and had gotten seasick again. So I thought I'd go the book one better and imagine myself becoming seasick every time I sat down to eat. By the next day I was dizzy and vomit-ing owing to labyrinthitis. My imaging had affected the organ of balance. I had to stay in bed for three or four days. My illness certainly mimicked the worst seasickness I've ever had. I strongly suggest that you never deliberately think negative thoughts about your body, even for a positive goal such as losing weight. The picture in your mind is likely to come much too true.

As I learned more about the mind-body link, I began to realize that I had become programmed to be seasick since I was five years old. That year I'd gone fishing with my father, had immediately gotten seasick, and presumed that I always would. My family and I still loved boating and fishing enough to keep trying year after year, but my discomfort cut into the fun. Just as many of my patients on chemotherapy get sick on the way to their oncologist's office, I would start to get seasick on the way to the boat. I decided I would have none of that, and through meditation I reprogrammed myself *not* to get sick. Next summer I was able to take my wife and children fishing several times without a trace of the problem. In fact, one of the trips was rather stormy, and I was so thrilled with my success that I kept us all out there until *they* started feeling a bit queasy.

To become exceptional in caring for the body, one must take stock of the beliefs one has about it, especially those so ingrained that they're normally unconscious. If a person can turn from predicting illness to anticipating recovery, the foundation for cure is laid.

I have a patient, a frail woman named Edith, who weighs all of eighty-five pounds. She told me, "I don't need you and your group. My mother always told me when I was a youngster, 'You're scrawny, but whatever happens, you'll always get over it. You'll live to be ninety-three, and then they'll have to run you over with a steamroller.' " Edith has survived a heart attack, a bleeding duodenal ulcer, the death of her husband, and breast cancer invading the chest wall. She is now alive more than half a dozen years after her surgery. Every time something happens, she hears her mother's words.

If we all programmed our children this way, we'd be creating survivors. As parents, we are, in a sense, our children's first hypnotists and can give them positive post-hypnotic suggestions.

Instead, negative conditioning is all too common. Over the years I've found that my patients tend to get the same diseases as their parents and to die at the same age. I think conditioning is at least as much a factor as genetic predisposition (I call it "psychological genetics"), because I've seen people change the scenario once they become aware of it. When a patient says resignedly, "I first learned about my cancer in March, I had a recurrence in March, and here it is March again," then has a second recurrence and dies within a month, you begin to see that there's more involved than genetics. Fatalism can be fatal. Too many people think they're doomed to reenact their parents' scripts. As a nurse told me after one of my lectures, "I think you may have saved my life. I've been waiting to die of cancer, since my mother has it and my father had it. It never occurred to me that I didn't have to have it."

I recently treated a patient named Henry, whose father used to tear the obituary page out of the newspaper, as well as any other page that had any mention of illness on it. Now Henry was confronted with cancer. His panic was incredible, but with a great deal of work we were able to bring him through surgery, and he has done beautifully. Yet the fear that was created because his parents never taught him to deal with illness was an enormous contrast with Arthur, who came to my office on the same day I initially examined Henry. Arthur was a Christian Scientist who came because his family wanted him to. Even though he had a much more serious condition than the other man, his fear was much less.

Psychological "genes" can be as helpful or as damaging as physical genes. I often see this when I have drawings from a parent and child who have each developed cancer. How incredible to see the similarity. One is often a duplicate of the other, although they were made years apart, neither patient having seen the other's drawing. A hopeless, helpless parent produces a hopeless, helpless child.

TARGET ORGANS

Psychological shaping in the formative years plays a large part in determining who will develop a serious illness. Its effects are even more specific, however. It often determines what disease will occur, and when and where it will appear.

Consider the experience of Lee, a psychologist who has helped conduct some of the ECaP workshops. His troubles began with a persistent hoarseness that was eventually diagnosed as carcinoma of the larynx. His physician told him that the "treatment of choice" was laryngectomy, adding, "The only things you won't be able to do are sing and scuba dive." This was intended as reassurance that the life changes would be inconsequential, but the doctor never asked what Lee's life was all about, and Lee never told him. Singing and scuba diving happened to be his favorite pastimes.

Lee was a nonsmoker, so the location of his tumor was unusual. As a result of his work with ECaP and his training as a psychologist, he realized there must be psychological factors at work. I suggested that his throat must have some special significance for him. Obviously, the ability to speak well was crucial to his profession.

We found that it went beyond the obvious. Lee's family was large and noisy, and often when the boy was talking loudly, his father put his hand around Lee's throat and squeezed, telling him, "Shut up, Lee. Shut up, Lee," in a husky, whispery voice just like Lee's esophageal speech now.

With much pain and work, Lee has overcome the effects of his childhood messages. After the operation, his physicians kept coming up with good reports, but intuitively he knew problems still existed, and finally the tests confirmed this. He developed a second cancer on his back, and then a third, lymphoma. Through all these trials he meekly went along with the "treatment of choice," until the last time, when he was told the most he could expect was another five years with chemotherapy.

Finally Lee spoke up for himself. He told his doctors he wanted more than a miserable few years on drugs. He wanted to beat the whole thing. He charted his own course of psychological readjustment and nutritional therapy. His oncologist told him he was "just chasing rainbows." Since the rainbow is a universal symbol of hope and life, that was just what he needed to hear. He is now alive and well, outdoing his specialist's prediction with no recurrence, despite abandoning standard medical treatment. Nevertheless, I don't necessarily recommend his approach to others. Not everyone is as strong as Lee, or can accomplish such profound change. For some his rigid nutritional program might become a burden, negating its benefits.

Lee's case is not unusual. Target organs—parts of the body

with special significance to the conflicts or losses in a person's life—are the most likely areas for disease to take root. Franz Alexander, the father of psychosomatic medicine, recognized this over forty years ago when he wrote: "There is much evidence that, just as certain pathological microorganisms have a specific affinity for certain organs, so also certain emotional conflicts possess specificities and accordingly tend to afflict certain internal organs." The discovery of oncogenes has been a great step forward in understanding cancer. Yet, if oncogenes are the sole cause, persons susceptible to cancer should develop many primary tumors at one time, in various parts of the body. Instead, they invariably develop cancer in only one area that is psychologically significant to them—the target organ.

Occasionally I get a chance to talk with psychiatrists, either as patients or at conferences. Many of them tell stories about patients' need for disease or the significance of target organs. One told me of a psychotic patient who became mentally well when he became physically ill and, as soon as the illness was over, became psychotic again. Another described a man who insisted he was pregnant and grew an enormous tumor of the urethra and prostate (the closest male equivalents of the womb), so that he *looked* pregnant.

I remember one woman in the hospital who gave me a positive statement when I asked her how she visualized her x-ray therapy. She said, "I see it as a golden beam of sunshine entering my body."

I told her, "Someone must have been here before me and explained all this to you."

She said, "Just the woman in the next bed." A woman with both hands in bandages was lying there. I talked to her and learned that six or seven years before she'd had a mesothelioma, was told she'd be dead in six months, made enormous spiritual changes in her life, and the disease had disappeared. I asked, "Why did you need *this* illness?" And she said, "I don't know."

We talked for a while, and she told me she had a lovely husband and two beautiful children, but at home there was no one to talk to about the incredible changes she had made in healing herself. And it was wonderful to be in the hospital. She had all the interns, nurses, and staff to talk to. I said, "Aha. Then that's why you're here with your hands wrapped up with these infections." And I said to her, "I'll find people for you to talk to. You go ahead and get well."

Women whose children die young or who have unhappy love relationships are especially vulnerable to breast or cervical diseases. One ECaP patient, who had lost two husbands to cancer, had uterine cancer and herpes zoster (shingles) in one of her breasts. I don't think it was a coincidence that, after two such losses, she developed diseases of two sex organs that would effectively keep other men away.

One of my breast-cancer patients was a perfect example, not only of this connection but also of the hope that comes from *realizing* the connection. Diana's son had lost his life in a hit-and-run accident, and she was making an enormous effort to track down the killer, since the police had botched the job and ruined the evidence. Her friends kept telling her that she was literally "killing herself." She became overweight and developed high blood pressure. Finally came the breast cancer that compounded her despair. As we talked, however, Diana came to realize that her own emotions and actions had contributed to her disease, and that by changing them she could contribute to her ability to get well. After she left the office, my nurse asked, "Didn't you tell her she has cancer?"

"Of course," I replied. "Why?"

"Because she was smiling on the way out."

Many patients already know something of this link and only require an open-minded doctor to be able to use the knowledge. As one said, "I was always considered spineless, and here I've developed multiple myeloma of my backbone." Or a woman involved in a stressful love affair with a married man says, "I was afraid I'd get cancer, and I knew if I did, it would be in the cervix." After seeing a man with cancer of the rectum, I asked him what had happened in the last year or two of his life. He said, "Nothing much." So I asked his daughter. She said she had married out of the family religion and her brother had run away from home. Later, while helping the man explore his attitudes in ECaP, one of the other members said, "That boy must have been some pain in the ass!" A multiple sclerosis patient whose household help left her with five young children to care for, lost the use of her right hand. She had just lost her right-hand man.

To an outsider a connection may sometimes seem farfetched, but only the patient can finally judge whether it's real or not. Having seen it happen time and time again, I've concluded that we sensitize the target organs of our bodies in a form of negative biofeedback.

PSYCHOLOGICAL PROFILE OF CANCER

In the second century A.D., Galen noted that melancholy people were more likely to get cancer than those with more sanguine dispositions. In the eighteenth and nineteenth centuries, many physicians realized that cancer tends to follow tragedy or crisis in a person's life, especially in those whom today we term depressed. Before the advent of modern psychology, however, there was little they could do to help their depressed patients change their outlook.

Despite the twentieth century's far-reaching discoveries about the mind, medicine has been strangely reluctant to apply them to a better understanding of cancer. Elida Evans, a student of Carl Jung, paved the way in 1926 with her *Psychological Study of Cancer,* but it went almost completely ignored. The copy I came across in the Yale Medical Library in the mid-1970s had been borrowed only six times in fifty years. The book clearly spells out the cancer risk incurred by the personality type for whom life's meaning comes entirely from people or things outside the self. When that connection is disrupted, illness follows. Evans concluded, "Cancer is a symbol, as most illness is, of something going wrong in the patient's life, a warning to him to take another road."

Today, thanks to further work by LeShan, Dr. Caroline Bedell Thomas, and others, we are able to sketch a fairly complete psychological profile of those people who are most likely to develop cancer.

The typical cancer patient, let's say a man, experienced a lack of closeness to his parents during childhood, a lack of the kind of unconditional love that could have assured him of his intrinsic value and ability to overcome challenges. As he grew up, he became strongly extraverted, but not so much from an innate attraction to others as from a dependency on them for validation of his own worth. Adolescence was an even harder time for this future cancer patient than for other teenagers. Difficulty in forming more than superficial friendships led to an excruciating loneliness and reinforcement of earlier feelings of inadequacy.

Such a person tends to view himself as stupid, clumsy, weak, and inept at social games or sports, despite real achievements that are often the envy of classmates. At the same time he may cherish a vision of the "real me," who is supremely gifted, destined to benefit the human race with vague but transcendent accomplishments. But this authentic self is carefully hidden in the belief that it would jeopardize the (subjectively) minimal acceptance and love that the person has received. He thinks, "If I act the way I really feel—childlike, brilliant, loving, and 'crazy'—I'll be rejected."

I gave one of my patients, a young woman named Adrienne, a copy of Gerald Jampolsky's book *Love Is Letting Go of Fear*. After she'd read it, she told me, "I was like this book. I was a 'flower child,' in love with the world, and my parents said, 'Grow up.' So I grew up and got cancer, and you walk in and say, 'Become a child.' " Adrienne went back to her authentic loving self and is well today. Loving doesn't mean one hasn't grown up. Being childlike is not childish.

At some time, however, usually in the late teens or early twenties, the patient-to-be falls in love, finds one or two close friends, gets a job that provides real satisfaction, or otherwise reaches some level of happiness based outside the self. He is unable to take any credit for this turn of events. It seems like pure luck, more than he deserves, but for the time being all is well. As an adult, he is still characterized by a poor self-image and passivity regarding his own needs, but he shows extreme devotion to the one other person, cause, or group that has become his life.

Sooner or later—it may be a few years, it may be decades —the external meaning vanishes. The friends move away, the job disappears or becomes less satisfying, the loved spouse leaves or dies. These changes happen to us all, and they are always painful, but to someone who has put all his eggs in one basket, the loss is disabling. Yet it usually doesn't appear to be. Others think he is "taking it remarkably well," but inside there is a hollowness. All the old feelings of unworthiness come flooding back, and all feeling of meaning in his life is lost.

The routine usually goes on. Having been a compulsive giver since childhood, the future cancer patient continues going through the motions with whoever remains in his life, until depleted and exhausted. Over and over again I hear friends and relatives say, "He was a saint. Why him?" The truth is that compulsively proper and generous people predominate among cancer patients because they put the needs of others ahead of their own. Cancer might be called the disease of nice people. They are "nice" by other people's standards, however. They are conditional lovers. They are giving only in order to receive love. If their giving is not rewarded, they are more vulnerable to illness than ever. It generally shows up within two years of the time when their psychological mainstay has disappeared.

The broadest, most complete picture has come from therapists working one-on-one with cancer patients and thus able to get an in-depth knowledge of the person's life as related to the disease. However, now there is also a rapidly increasing body of experimental evidence, focusing on specific aspects of the profile.

By using a simple psychological test on a large group of women, some of whom had cervical cancer, Arthur Schmale was able to pick out 36 of the 51 who had malignancies (already diagnosed but unknown to him), by looking for hopelessness and a recent emotional loss. Other research groups have since gotten even better results. Marjorie and Claus Bahnson have developed a questionnaire that is 88 percent accurate in identifying those who turn out to have a biopsy-confirmed cancer. Most of these psychological tests are now more accurate than physicians' physical exams. By the same token, the receptionist in my office is a pretty good diagnostician, basing her suppositions merely upon her contact with the new patient.

Some of the most valuable work has been done by Dr. Caroline Bedell Thomas of Johns Hopkins University Medical School. Beginning in 1946, she took personality profiles of 1,337 medical students, then surveyed their mental and physical health every year for decades after graduation. Her goal was to find psychological antecedents of heart disease, high blood pressure, mental illness, and suicide. She included cancer in the study for the sake of comparison, because she originally thought it would have no psychological component. However, the data showed a "striking and unexpected" result: the traits of those who developed cancer were almost identical to those of the students who later committed suicide. Almost all the cancer patients had throughout their lives been restricted in expressing emotion, especially aggressive emotions related to their own needs. She also found that, using only the drawings they made as one of the tests, she could predict what parts of their bodies would develop cancer.

Certain other diseases also stem from a lifelong pattern of self-denial. In chronic rheumatoid arthritis, for example, there is often a *conscious* restriction of one's own achievements. When I mentioned this to my mother, who has arthritis, she agreed: "Yes, that's me. I've belonged to many organizations, and I would work my way up to be vice-president, but when I was offered the presidency, I would say, 'No, I'm too involved with my family. I have to refuse.'"

It's important for a patient to understand the lifelong pattern, but for the immediate purpose—getting well—the problem must be put in terms that can be dealt with now. In most cases, this involves a recognition of conflict. For cancer patients it usually means finding out how the needs of others, seen as the only ones that count, are used to cover up one's own.

Often a real power struggle develops. I saw this most clearly and tragically in the case of Norma, an ECaP member with an abusive husband. Her disease started to disappear as she became more "self-caring." Then her husband developed heart disease and was hospitalized. Norma was faced with a choice. Rather than force her husband to choose between growing with her or fostering his illness, she chose to return to her old self. He resumed his abuse and got well, while she went home to die, telling the rest of the group there was to be no "funny business"—i.e., no attempts to change her mind—if we came to visit her.

Each of us has more or less the same choices. Norma's husband could have learned to love, or she could have asserted herself and gone on to live. But old patterns, though painful, are easier. Change is difficult, uncomfortable, and frightening. That's how we know we're changing.

It is often extraordinarily hard for the compulsive giver to stop, to say no without feeling guilty. Many of my female patients have come to group meetings saying, "I'll do anything to get well." Then I outline our program, including time for exercise and meditation, and they say, "Oh, but then dinner will be late." A patient named Sharon told us her husband's secretary had left, so she "had" to go in and work for him until he could find a replacement. The trouble was she hated the job. I told her, "You can't survive cancer if you get up every morning thinking how you hate what you'll be doing all day." Still it took her two or three months to, as she put it, "give her husband notice."

When individuals think about saying no, the thing that most often helps them do it is the sense of a time limit in their lives. If you knew you had a day to live, would you spend three hours lying in the x-ray department waiting for a test to be done? Hell, no. You'd say, "Take me back to my room. This is the last twenty-four hours of my life, and I'm not going to spend one-eighth of it in the x-ray department." Then they'll probably get the test done in five minutes.

I tell all my patients to make their choices based on what would feel right if they knew they were going to die in a day, a week, or a year. That's one way of giving people an immediate awareness of how they feel, even if they have never paid any attention to feelings. We don't have the luxury of five years of psychoanalysis when someone may not live that long. We have to begin change immediately, and the best way is by asking what you'd want to do with this short period of time.

INDIVIDUAL REACTIONS

Any psychological picture of cancer can only be a general one, of course, and examples from other people can only serve as guideposts. Though the broad features are the same, the specifics are different for each individual. However, many of our cancer patients are astonished when other cancer patients outline their personalities and life stories without ever having met them before. That can be a key motivating factor. The patient may think, "Wow! If you know all that, I guess I'd better change my life." The work of uncovering conflicts is the most important job facing the patient, for when the outer choices match the inner desires, energy formerly tied up in contradictions becomes available for healing.

My job as a physician is not only to find the right treatment but to help the patient find an inner reason for living, resolve conflicts, and free healing energy. Although the mind is incredibly powerful, it often takes something equally powerful to turn it on. That's why I ask patients to mobilize their faith in everything they can possibly believe in. Patients who want to get well through the doctor alone or God alone are minimizing their chances. More often than not, such people are really thinking, "I'm not so sure I want to survive, so I'll limit myself to the comfortable choices." The frequency of passive suicide remains unknown, but it's definitely a factor.

The one crucial question is what approach will work for each person. Never underestimate the value of the truth, even if it's a shock. I remember a patient who was in congestive heart failure, not taking her medicine, smoking like a chimney, and then coming to me for a gallbladder operation. I asked her, "Did you come here to have me kill you?"

The question surprised her. She said, "Nobody has talked to me like that since I gave up psychotherapy." I just explained that, before I could deal with her gallbladder, I had to deal with her depression and try to give her a reason for living.

I recently saw a patient with a brain tumor that had already progressed to the point of causing seizures. She was trying to decide whether to have it surgically removed or treat it only with a nutritional program. A friend had asked her to talk to me, since her regular doctors were all angry at her for shying away from aggressive treatment of this critical illness. I sat and talked with her until we got to the root of the problem —the fact that she was very depressed, with no great desire to go on living. Therefore, it was easier for her just to change her diet a little. This would cause her no great discomfort, and if she died it would be no great loss as far as she was concerned. My effort, then, was to show her how to make her life interesting enough to continue living. Then she would be in a position to choose modern techniques for dealing with the emergency, as well as to change her outlook thoroughly for the future.

I recommend that patients do *not* reject standard medical techniques, at least as one option. Most people are simply not strong enough to "leave their troubles to God," that is, heal themselves through finding peace of mind and developing a clear conscience. Drugs and surgery buy time, and may cure, while patients work to change their lives.

Soon after we'd set up ECaP, I was interviewed by the *Midnight Globe* tabloid. The resulting article was very fair and the quotations accurate, but I was upset by the headline: "Surgeon Says Mind Can Cure Cancer." I thought it was simplistic and misleading. The more I worked with patients, however, the more I came to see that the statement was correct. Now I consider those omnipresent supermarket newspapers to be important medical journals. (I say this tongue mostly in cheek.) The mind *can* cure cancer, but that doesn't mean it's easy.

The paradox is wonderfully expressed by an old Sufi story. A stranger comes upon a man on his hands and knees under a street lamp in front of his house. He's looking for his keys, and the stranger gets down on all fours to help him. After a time, the stranger asks, "Where exactly did you drop them?"

"In my house," comes the reply.

Exasperated, the stranger asks, "Then why are you looking out here?"

"Because it's dark in the house."

The light is better in our conscious minds, but we must look for healing in the dark unconscious. The doctor works in the light. He is verbal and logical. The patient's world may be dark, but there *are* sources of illumination. Within each of us is a spark. Call it a divine spark if you will, but it is there and can light the way to health. There are no incurable diseases, only incurable people.

4

*In the long run . . . no conscious will can ever replace
the life instinct.*

—CARL JUNG, *Late Thoughts*

The Will to Live

One of my patients, as soon as she was diagnosed as having cancer, went home and donated all her clothes to Goodwill Industries. More clearly than anything she ever said, this act showed her belief that the disease would inevitably kill her, so she might as well give up without a fight.

For many people, "You have cancer" are the three most dreaded words in our language. Those who hear them experience many emotions, which often change as people accept the news and deal with it. Some of these feelings may remain buried in the unconscious, and it's essential to bring them into the patient's conscious awareness.

Initially, the diagnosis is always handled with some degree of denial. This allows a person to accept it over a period of time. Sometimes patients are more depressed six months later than when they first hear the bad news, because it may take that long to truly hear what they have been told. Some persons seem to disbelieve the diagnosis, going on with their lives as though nothing is wrong. Usually they are simply denying their emotions: internally they are coming apart, but they refuse to reveal their feelings, perhaps because of early parental messages, such as "Don't tell the neighbors your troubles." That is a sure way to self-destruct. Performing for the sake of others destroys you.

A small number may act almost psychotic, really believing that nothing has happened to them. If a person can maintain that kind of abnormal denial, then cancer is not an emotional stress. But the majority cannot.

Others seem to accept the truth, yet refuse to admit it on a deeper level. These are often the ones who submit to treatment but never commit themselves wholeheartedly to trying to get well. One of my patients declined to join ECaP with the explanation "I haven't told my children I have cancer, so how can I appear in a group? I might meet someone I know." To many people, it's less painful in the short run to keep up a false front than to confront the terror of a life-threatening illness. Knowing the truth yet refusing to admit it prevents an effective response. Sharing one's fears and problems leads to relief and healing within the body. Knowing what you are fighting and how to fight are the keys. Denial may be better than stoicism or despair but it is not the best approach. I try to carefully convert deniers into fighters.

As we've seen in the previous chapter, those who develop cancer have often felt a sense of despair about their lives for months or years. After the diagnosis, they may feel this even more painfully, sometimes withdrawing from all human contact. They may also see their impending death as a sort of sacrifice or martyrdom. These are the ones who refuse to spend money on treatment because they feel they must save it for other people's needs, such as their children's college education. Some simply have never done anything for themselves and don't "know how." Others are trading their illness for conditional love and may even, in a sense, die to gain love.

Many cancer patients experience a flood of self-pity, an attitude of "Why me?" This is usually linked to strong feelings of anger, only some of which are conscious. The patient wonders why he, instead of someone else, has been afflicted with a predisposition to cancer. Hence many people get furious with God, as well as with the physician—the messenger who brought the bad news. Oddly enough, only a few express rage against the cigarette industry, the pesticide industry, the food-additive industry, the nuclear-power industry, and other external sources of malignancy. In the case of smoking, patients tend to realize that they took the risk themselves because they were unhappy, and thus get angry with family members and others who, they feel, made them unhappy. While the typical patient may ask, "Why me, Lord?" the exceptional patient says, as one ECaP member did, "Try me, Lord."

I want to emphasize that *all* emotions are justified at this stage and must be expressed. Much of the anger is well founded. Cancer's complex causes aren't all in the mind. Genes and carcinogens are important factors, and it's worthwhile to work toward genetic cures and environmental sanity. But some whose parents had cancer or who have been heavily exposed to carcinogens still don't come down with the disease. Cigarette smokers who are emotionally well adjusted or who eat a healthy diet high in vitamin A have less lung cancer than those who are depressed or eat poorly. To balance our research into cancer's molecular seeds, we need to learn about the state of mind and body that prevents the seeds from growing.

Moreover, patients often concentrate on the obvious external targets while more personal angers that are harder to acknowledge remain hidden and increase their susceptibility to illness. For those who already have cancer, the psychological aspects of the disease are the crucial ones. We can't change the past—our parents and our exposure to carcinogens—but we can change ourselves and thus our future. As one of my patients said, "Cancer isn't a sentence, it's just a word."

When I began ECaP, I experienced tremendous amounts of this anger. The first group of patients had never had a chance to express it, and they all came angry to the first meetings. Initially this made it hard for me to talk to other doctors about my work. I heard so much anger at physicians that when I left the meetings I was mad at doctors, too. For a while I told every colleague I met, "You're a typical doctor." They knew this was a derogatory statement. Fortunately, my partners asked me what was happening, and I realized I was taking home my patients' anger, because I was the only one there to absorb it. Now the more experienced ECaP members also help the newcomers work through their rage.

I'm not saying that anger at the externals should be suppressed—just the opposite. Patients must be encouraged to express all their angers, resentments, hatreds, and fears. These emotions are signs that we care to the utmost when our lives are threatened. Time after time, research has shown that people who give vent to their negative emotions survive adversity better than those who are emotionally constricted. Among patients with spinal-cord injuries, those who express strong grief and anger make more progress in rehabilitation than those with a more stoical attitude. Mothers who show great distress after giving birth to a deformed infant give the child better care than those who seem to take the misfortune calmly. In a study of people living near Three Mile Island, Dr. Andrew Baum found that those who showed their rage and fear suffered far less from stress and psychological problems than those who took a "rational" approach. Unexpressed feelings depress your immune response.

Some cancer patients also experience strong feelings of guilt. They blame themselves, just as many children who get sick think their illness is a punishment for being bad. Although not ideal, this attitude is not entirely destructive, for it often leads to a more realistic sense of participation in the onset of disease. In fact, a large amount of research on people who've suffered catastrophe has proven that those who feel they contributed to it (even if they did not) tend to get over the trauma more easily than those who feel totally helpless. This holds true for such tragedies as rape, earthquakes, and floods, as well as sickness. For example, if a woman who has been raped can think, no matter what the circumstances, "It wouldn't have happened if I'd been more careful, if I had learned to protect myself," she can reduce her sense of powerlessness and plan to make herself less vulnerable in the future. Researchers have found that such an attitude enables people to accept human evil and natural disaster without believing that life is devoid of beauty or meaning.

Using a battery of psychological tests, Leonard Derogatis discovered in 1979 that breast-cancer patients who felt and freely expressed much anger, fear, depression, and guilt lived far longer than patients who showed little of these emotions. Those who died within a year had relied heavily on repression, denial, and other psychological defenses. The hostility that the survivors vented on their physicians led to the conclusion, mentioned in Chapter 1, that they formed "poor" doctor-patient relationships. Derogatis used rigorous statistical controls to exclude physical differences between the short-term and long-term survivors. His work stands as excellent scientific support for a group of researchers nearly three decades earlier, who were "impressed by the polite, apologetic, almost painful acquiescence of patients with rapidly progressive disease as contrasted to the more expressive and sometimes bizarre personalities" of those who lived longer.

THE FOUR QUESTIONS

Before I can help patients choose treatment, I must learn about their attitudes toward themselves and their disease. It is especially important to gauge the strength of their will to live, and then to strengthen it by getting them to express their anger, fear, and other emotions. As Norman Cousins wrote in his *Anatomy of an Illness,*

The will to live is not a theoretical abstraction, but a physiologic reality with therapeutic characteristics.

◆ ◆ ◆

Not every illness can be overcome. But many people allow illness to disfigure their lives more than it should. They cave in needlessly. They ignore and weaken whatever powers they may have for standing erect. There is always a margin within which life can be lived with meaning and even with a certain measure of joy, despite illness.

At first a patient's emotions and attitudes may not be fully accessible to consciousness. To retrieve them I've found that we need to explore the answers to four basic questions.

1. *Do you want to live to be a hundred?*

Most people won't answer without some hypothetical guarantee of health. They don't instinctively take the responsibility for making all their years worthwhile. A few years ago gerontologist Ken Dychtwald asked hundreds of people, "How old do you want to be before you die?" A majority didn't want to live past sixty or sixty-five, because they assumed their lives then would be devoid of play, sex, independence, or meaning, and filled with problems. The elderly, however, tended to want more years, and women generally wanted more years than men.

This question always leads to others, such as "Do you love yourself enough to take care of your body and mind?" The answer is contained in your lifestyle. Do you eat moderately, avoiding too much sugar, caffeine, and fat? Are there plenty of fresh fruits and vegetables in your diet? Do you avoid most processed, additive-laden foods? Do you smoke? Do you eat a good breakfast and get adequate rest? Do you exercise? Are you self-motivated? (Most centenarians have been self-employed for much of their lives.) Do you seek activities that give you joy and satisfaction?

The answers all depend on whether or not you feel in control of your life and thus whether you look forward to the future with hope or with fear. One ECaP member, a wonderful woman named Shirley, joined the group at the age of ninety-two. Once, when everyone was talking about how afraid they were of cancer, pain, dying, and so on, I asked her, "Shirley, what are you afraid of?"

She said, "Driving on the parkway at night." That put the other members' fears to rest, because she has lived through everything they're still afraid of, except death. Remember if you decide to live to be 100 loved ones may die before you. It takes courage to survive and be "the last apple on the tree," as one of my patients said.

2. What happened to you in the year or two before your illness?

This question, along with tools such as the Holmes-Rahe stress scale, explores the short-term psychological predisposing factors discussed in Chapter 3. Inevitably, it also leads back to the long-term conditioning factors that determine how a person reacts to the recent events. It's essential to consider internal stresses, too, such as an identity crisis or the giving up of one of youth's cherished dreams. We must also consider how the patient reacted to the crisis. Did he or she openly grieve, rejoice, and face the challenge, or try to be calm and stoical?

3. What does the illness mean to you?

If cancer, for example, automatically means death, then the patient has a problem that must be solved before dealing with the disease itself. Such a meaning is programmed and reinforced by silence. When the adults in a family say, "We don't talk about that," or a parent says, "You get whatever your sister gets, and whatever happens to your sister happens to you," when the sister dies of cancer the siblings believe there is no hope for them. Without frank acceptance, death, like sex, becomes an embarrassment. The husband who only tells his wife over and over, "Don't die," or "You're going to get well," no matter how extensive the disease, prevents her from sharing her fears and hinders her efforts to face death openly. In such an atmosphere, the patient is cast into the outer darkness without love or any way to share emotions. On the other hand, if the disease means a challenge, formidable but not invincible —then the patient has a basis for dealing with it.

This question is useful, but actions and expectations are often even more revealing. Jennifer had been entered in a hospice program by her doctor, who expected her to die within six months. But she kept on living. When the hospice staff asked if she looked forward to spring, she said, "Oh, yes, I love to watch the flowers come up." They asked if she liked summer. "Very much." Fall? "Oh, I just love the leaves changing color." Even winter? "Yes, the snow." Eventually the hospice personnel told her they had to stop coming. They would return when she was ready to die. She became a "hospice dropout" and joined one of our ECaP groups.

When winter approached, however, Jennifer told me, "I don't think I'm going to be buying any winter clothes." This indicated that perhaps she was getting ready to die.

Then she came to one of our meetings wearing a lovely winter suit. I said, "Aha! I see you decided to buy some winter clothes."

"No," she said, "I just brought some down from the attic." To me that said she'd made a compromise. She was saying, "Let's see how the winter goes. I'm not going to invest in it, but I'll give it a try."

Another cancer patient I know, named Matt, went to his physician one day looking awful and came home looking fine. His family asked, "Gee, what did the doctor do?"

Matt said, "Oh, he gave me my allergy shot." This let him know that the doctor expected him to live through the spring, and his body responded.

4. *Why did you need the illness?*

Like the previous two questions, this one helps the patient understand the psychological needs that the disease may meet. Sickness gives people "permission" to do things they would otherwise be inhibited from doing. It can make it easier to say no to unwelcome burdens, duties, jobs, or the demands of other people. It can serve as permission to do what one has always wanted but has always been "too busy" to start. It can allow a person to take time off to reflect, meditate, and chart a new course. It can serve as an excuse for failure. It can make it easier to request and accept love, speak your feelings, or otherwise be more honest. Even a cold has a meaning. Often its message is "You've been working too hard. Go home and nurture yourself." Remember we are brought up on "sick days," not "health days." Take days to meet your needs and you won't need an illness.

Since physical illness usually brings sympathy from friends and relatives, it can be a way of gaining love, or nurturing. It can become a patient's only way of relating to the world, the only control one has over life. Gladys, a patient of mine who'd had a chronic intestinal inflammation for some fifty years, learned to manipulate her whole family this way. I met her after she developed cancer. The family looked sicker than she did, because she had some family member awake to wait on her twenty-four hours a day. Even when they hired a nurse to care for her, Gladys would awaken the family and let the nurse sleep. Over and over she developed severe pains at home, which mysteriously disappeared each time she was admitted to the hospital. Nearly every weekend she would have those who were not home during the week in the emergency room with her to help evaluate her recurrent chest pains. Thus those who worked during the week got their share. She was constantly asking someone to hand her a glass of water or a tissue, even when what she wanted was only inches away.

After I got to know Gladys, I gave her Arnold Hutschnecker's *The Will to Live*. The next morning when I returned on my rounds, she said I'd forgotten something—the book. The message was clear: "Please don't try to teach me to give up my illness, because it's the only way I can relate to people." Learning to love was frightening.

I kept trying to reach Gladys, and she said I was the only doctor who ever gave her hope. Truthfully I think I was the only one who continued to care for her without being worn out by constant manipulation, which included side effects to every medication I recommended. I learned to let her do much of the talking, then recommend things that fit her belief system. Then I would always get the credit and be called a wonderful doctor.

Finally, during one of her phone calls, I told her I had a new drug that would cure her cancer. I asked her to come to the office, since it had to be given by injection. I did this after explaining my plan to the family and asking them to watch Gladys's reaction. I was trying to save *them* from being the victims of *her* illness. She made an appointment for Friday, but on that day she called to postpone it for a week because the weather was bad. Next Friday she couldn't get a ride, and the week after that she had to go shopping. In short, Gladys never returned to my office, although she tried to maintain our relationship by phone or at the hospital, where I didn't have the drug. I took this approach only for the family's sake, since I knew she would refuse the offer. Her family then had the option of going along in the old pattern or refusing to be victimized any longer.

It's important to realize that we can't force others to change, we can only help them to change themselves. I have had two male patients much like Gladys, both with extensive cancers. I said to each of them, "I'll guarantee you a cure of your cancer if you leave your family business," which both found very stressful but meaningful, and which would give the family many benefits in the event of the man's death. Each man said exactly the same thing: "I'll have to go home and think about it."

A cancer patient was advised by his surgeon to sell his business, because the surgeon felt he was terminal. He did, and got well. One day I encountered him in the hospital hallway. He was yelling at his surgeon—because now he was well but had no business. I explained that he'd been given the right advice for the wrong reason. He'd been encouraged to quit because statistics said he would soon die, whereas the reduced stress and more enjoyable life had in fact led to his recovery.

My purpose is not to judge these patients' motives, but to bring them out into the open. Then the family knows when a person doesn't really want to change, and can work on the conflict with love, and meet its needs too.

Throughout our lives we're trained to associate sickness with rewards. We get to stay in bed and relax. People send us cards and flowers. Friends visit and tell us they love us. Parents and spouses bring us chicken soup and read to us. I remember a patient named Myrna telling me that the happiest times in her childhood were when she was sick, because then her father would sit on her bed and hold her hand. Her experience is far from unique. As children we get to stay home from school, and as adults we get a paid respite from work. If we stay healthy, we have to either show up every day or *pretend* to be sick. We should be able to call up and say, "I want to stay well, so today I'm taking a health day."

Even our insurance system rewards illness by penalizing those who take care of themselves. If payments reflected our commitment to health instead of statistical assumptions based on age, family history, and a cursory physical, we could give people more of an incentive to take charge of their health. We should establish certain basic requirements—controlling weight, not smoking, and so on. When those are met for a minimum fee, all medical expenses would be covered. Those who meet none of the requirements would have to pay much larger premiums. Cigarette and liquor taxes could also be set aside for a national health-insurance fund to keep those who work at their health from having to pay the bills of those who don't.

Those who try to get patients to understand how their own actions have contributed to illness are often criticized for "blaming the victim." This attitude misses the point. All people eventually die even when they've done some beautiful things. And even when a person's lifestyle obviously contributed to disease, guilt is not a productive way of relating to the effects of the past. No doctor should ever encourage a patient to take on this additional burden. Illness and the prospect of death are not seen as failures but as motivators.

However, most illnesses do have a psychological component, and a realization of one's *participation* and responsibility in the disease process is entirely different from blame or guilt. Of course few ever really want a life-threatening sickness, but it usually functions as a message to change or gives patients something they are not getting from their lives. As Carl Simonton has said, "I believe we develop our diseases for honorable reasons. It's our body's way of telling us that our needs—not just our body's needs but our emotional needs, too—are not being met, and the needs that are fulfilled through our illnesses are important ones."

It cannot be overemphasized that this last and most important question—Why did you need this illness?—must be asked constructively, not as a way of saying, "Look what a mess you've made of your life." It is intended to help patients realize that the emotional needs met by illness are all valid. Then, when the needs are accepted, a person can move on to satisfy them in constructive ways, without the disease.

William James wrote, "The greatest discovery of my generation is that human beings, by changing the inner attitudes of their minds, can change the outer aspects of their lives." Years of experience have taught me that cancer and indeed nearly all diseases are psychosomatic. This may sound strange to people accustomed to thinking that psychosomatic ailments are not truly "real," but, believe me, they are. The new concept is not a cop-out, but rather a source of tremendous hope. David Bohm, the physicist, suggests the word "soma-signifi-cance" as a better way of thinking of the relationship. The body knows only what the mind tells it. To accept some of the responsibility for disease, to realize that one has participated, is actually a very positive step. If one has taken part in getting sick, one can also take part in getting well.

However, as I'll discuss in more detail later, getting well isn't the main objective. That can set you up for failure. If you set a physical goal, then you may fail, but if you make peace of mind your goal, you *can* achieve it. My message is peace of mind, not curing cancer, blindness, or paraplegia. In achieving peace of mind, cancer may be healed, sight may be restored, and paralysis may disappear. All of these things may occur through peace of mind, which creates a healing environment in the body. Anyone who is willing to work at it can achieve it, and the first step is understanding—realistically, without guilt or self-pity—how the mind has contributed to the body's ills. This understanding can show you how you must change to be at peace with yourself.

MESSAGES FROM THE UNCONSCIOUS

The mind and body communicate constantly with each other, but most of this communication is on an unconscious level. Therefore, the doctor must ask the patient about his attitudes but must not take all the answers at face value. What seems like a strong will to live may actually be a surface re-solve, a performance, rather than a true inner connection to the life force. It's necessary to get beyond the verbal, conscious level to make sure that what the patient says is what he really feels. The surest way to do this is by examining images from his unconscious mind.

These images surface spontaneously in dreams, which sometimes can be used to diagnose physical illness, as Carl Jung was able to do. However, the process of inferring somatic facts from mental images is so complex and often involves such seemingly far-fetched connections that even Jung declined to discuss it, for fear of having his work rejected. Fostering and interpreting diagnostic and curative dreams was essential to the methods of ancient Greek and Egyptian healing temples and was practiced by Hippocrates and Galen, but today it is a lost art just beginning to be restudied by a few psychologists. It is not yet a tool that most doctors can use.

However, some spontaneous dreams are relatively easy to interpret. Often a patient and I can understand a dream by discussing it together. Sandy had such a dream when she developed breast cancer during her second marriage. She saw three roads ahead of her: one gray and black with everyone carrying a heavy bundle, a second road filled with many colors and active, cheerful people, and a third, which she couldn't see clearly. After drawing a picture of the dream and talking it over in the group, she realized that the first road represented her cancer as a burden and bringing despair, the second represented it as a challenge to live and develop, and the third represented the choice she would have to make. She chose the path of life, and as she grew, her cancer shrank. She responded well to therapy and was "reborn" as a new person. She shared her experience by writing articles and eventually went back to school and now has a new career and her health.

The easiest dreams to understand are those with self-explanatory images or those which the dreamer spontaneously knows the meaning of. One patient with breast cancer dreamed her head was shaved and the word cancer was written on her scalp. She woke knowing she had brain metastases. There were no physical signs or symptoms until three weeks later, when the dream diagnosis was confirmed. I once had a dream during a time when I was having certain symptoms that might have been due to cancer. In my dream I was a member of a group whose other members all had cancer, but I was pointed out as not having it. Tests later verified what the dream had communicated.

One day in the operating room I was discussing dreams and a nurse recounted one of the "direct insight" dreams. She had been very sick for several weeks, and no one could figure out what was wrong. Then one night she had a dream in which a shellfish opened, a worm stood up inside it, and an old woman pointed at the worm and said, "That's what's wrong with you." The nurse woke up knowing she had hepatitis, which was confirmed by subsequent tests.

Such direct dreams often give information that medical tests can't. One leukemia patient, who had recently had a bone-marrow aspiration whose results were normal, nevertheless dreamed of termites eating away at the foundation of her house. We encouraged her to imagine exterminators being brought in during her meditations, but she then dreamed of maggots eating potatoes at her feet. She died in three weeks. Her mind knew what the tests didn't.

Often, however, dream interpretation is difficult, even for an experienced psychotherapist. The meaning of the symbols often depends on emotions or events in the patient's life that may be hidden from consciousness. Dreams can be explored on two levels. The first is the level of personal meanings, which can almost always be worked out with the patient. The other is the deeper, unconscious level of symbols and myths, which is more problematic. Anyone who takes the time can explore his or her own dreams on the first level. For this there are several excellent books that can serve as guides, including Gail Delaney's *Living Your Dreams,* Ann Faraday's *The Dream Game,* and Patricia Garfield's *Creative Dreaming.* Jung's techniques are discussed in "The Meaning in Dreams and Dreaming" by Maria F. Mahoney.

Fortunately, there is a simpler, more reliable way to reveal unconscious beliefs. The doctor merely asks the patient to draw a picture. I give all new patients the following instructions:

1. On a white sheet of paper, held vertically, draw a picture of yourself, your treatment, your disease, and your white blood cells eliminating the disease. Please have all colors of the rainbow, brown, black, and white available to you, and use crayons.
2. On a separate sheet of white paper, held horizontally, draw another picture or scene in color using crayons.
3. You may also choose to draw an additional picture of your home and family, as well as additional images

(such as a tree, boat, or bird, etc.) that may call forth
further significant material from the unconscious.
Pictures relating to conflicts or choices, such as a job or
impending surgery, may also be important.

Such drawings bypass verbal deceptions and get to the
universal symbolic language of the unconscious. What we say
is often a cover-up, because we're all trained in language and
use it, consciously or not, to conceal things that disturb us. But
when we communicate in visual images, we tell the truth,
because we can't manipulate the language as well. This is a
language of the collective unconscious. The patient's and doctor's appearance, religion, race, culture, and language are all
unimportant, for the archetypal pictures inside us are all the
same and have the same meanings.

Of course, it is important to know some specifics about a
patient's background, because conscious statements involving
them may be made in the drawing. For example, if a patient
draws himself wearing a black suit and says he chose that color
simply because he was wearing a black suit that day, then you
can't infer anything about his emotional state from the symbolism of the color.

When these aspects of the drawing have been dealt with,
however, it remains a vital window on the unconscious. Susan
R. Bach, the Jungian therapist who developed a systematic
approach to the interpretation of spontaneous pictures, has
written:

The study of such spontaneous material could give us a
glimpse into the psyche-soma relation comprehended as the
oldest and best married couple on this earth, serving conjointly
the life and health of the individual, each in its own right, with its
own mode of expression and its own laws.
Further study and deeper understanding made me aware
that the somatic side is equally reflected in the pictorial images of
dreams, in the work of artists, in basic motifs of fairy tales, in
heroic figures of mythology, down to prehistoric paintings of early
man. They can be comprehended as an expression of man as a
whole.

I've found that analysis of these drawings is one of a doctor's most accurate aids to prognosis. When there's time, I even use the approach in the emergency room. When a child with abdominal pain, for example, just draws her head with her eyes looking around with an expression that says, "I don't like this place," it's a good bet there's nothing seriously wrong with her abdomen. I remember a young man who colored his abdomen green, even though every note on his chart said, "Operate." Green is a natural, healthy color, and the drawing indicated that the trouble spots were the man's head, genitals, and one foot. The drawing represented an emotional problem, a sexual problem, and a foot that he had injured. We waited, and he recovered without surgery. We learned later that the abdominal pain was due to a drug reaction, not disease. This and similar experiences have led me to think of myself as a Jungian surgeon.

A child in my office shared for the first time with her parents a dream that told her she would have cancer in a year in her right leg. She told her sister not to tell the parents as they would only worry for a year. She began to draw one-legged teddy bears and a year later had an amputation for a sarcoma of her right leg. The story came out because I created a safe environment for this discussion as we shared the families' drawings.

When combined with other psychological tests, mental imagery often is more useful than laboratory tests in assessing the patient's prospects. Work done by the Simontons, Jeanne Achterberg and G. Frank Lawlis compared the predictive value of psychological factors and blood chemistry in 126 patients with extensive cancer. Virtually every psychological test showed a statistical relationship to one or more blood components. The patients who did most poorly were those who were very dependent on others—such as the doctor—for motivation and esteem, who used psychological defenses to deny their condition, and who visualized their bodies as having little power to fight the disease. Compared with patients who did well, those whose disease progressed fastest were more conformist to sex-role stereotypes and developed images that were more concrete and less creative or symbolic. The re-

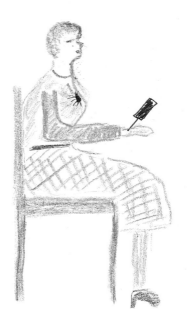

Here we see someone sitting down on the job and only giving half of herself (the side view) to the problem. She depicted her disease as an insect, a negative symbol. The treatment is black, bringing despair, and it is not entering her body, showing nonacceptance.

This drawing suggests a very negative outcome if the individual doesn't change. Trying to look on the bright side (to the right, or east) isn't enough to turn things around.

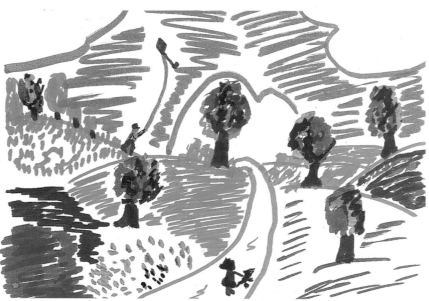

Linda, who is mentioned on page 40, is the woman in the center. She portrayed herself in orange, a color that denotes change. The purple kite reveals her readiness for a peaceful, spiritual transition, but her husband is holding onto the kite. Realizing that he depended on her and was not prepared for her death, she decided not to die and began chemotherapy. Finally Linda's husband told her, "Honey, I've cut the string. It's all right for you to go." She said, "I'm going to die on Thursday at two o'clock when the children get here from California." In the hospital I asked her, "Are there any questions you have about dying?" She laughed and said, "I've never died before, so I don't know what questions to ask." She left her body peacefully at the time of her choosing.

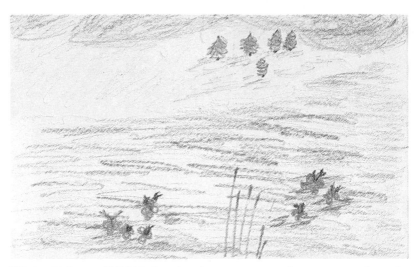

This drawing by my wife Bobbie shows how the unconscious reveals processes in our lives. The five trees represent our five children, and as you can see, one of them is out of line. The solution lies in the seven water lilies at the bottom, grouped four and three. At the time of the drawing, two of our sons, Jon and Stephen, were away at college, in Chicago and Denver. Jeff was trying to decide what to do about school. The group of four symbolized Bobbie and me and the twins, our two youngest children, remaining at home. The group of three showed Jon, Stephen, and now Jeff, away. When we looked at the drawing, we knew Jeff had already made his decision.

Six cattails separate the two groups of our family, and six weeks to the day after Bobbie made the drawing Jeff left to join his brother and attend school in Denver.

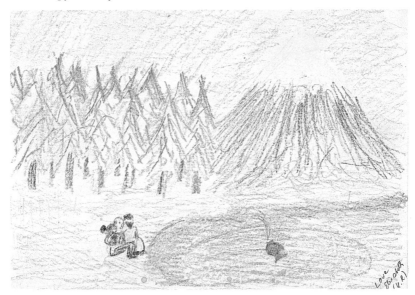

I made this drawing at a workshop given by Elisabeth Kübler-Ross. Note the snow-covered mountaintop (white on white, signifying something covered up) and the fish out of water (the spiritual symbol out of its element).

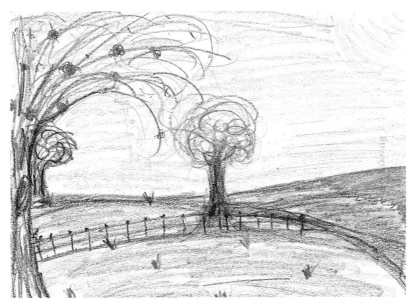

Two trees are seen separated by a fence and one tree seems to be straddling the fence. Trees often represent the entire psyche and/or soma. In this case the two trees on either side of the fence represent a couple kept apart by some issue, symbolized by the fence. One tree is bearing fruit. It stands for the one wage-earner in the relationship, and it is almost out of the picture.

The issue to be dealt with was the fact that the wife was earning money while the husband was not, and was not making any attempt to. This woman had to choose whether to leave, continue the status quo, or stay while refusing to accept her husband's behavior. Her indecision is represented by the tree that appears to be on both sides of the fence.

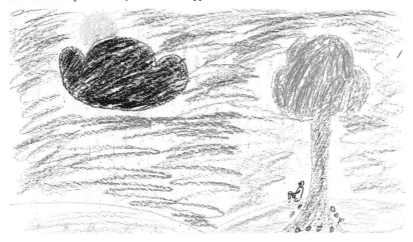

This patient drew himself as a small, forlorn figure sitting under a protecting tree, which symbolized his wife helping him. Black clouds are in the future, and the number of fallen fruit represented his time left. Since people are capable of change, we always work at altering negative images, but often there is an inner knowing, which when shared relieves the patient of a burden.

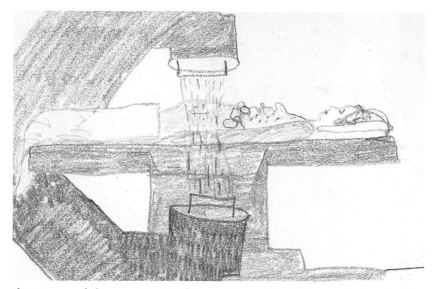

This picture symbolizes a positive attitude to x-ray therapy. The whole person is shown in a blue machine (a healthy color), with purple and yellow (spiritual and celestial) rays entering her body only where the disease is. The patient anticipates a good therapeutic result without side effects. The image shows an acceptance of therapy on both the conscious and unconscious levels.

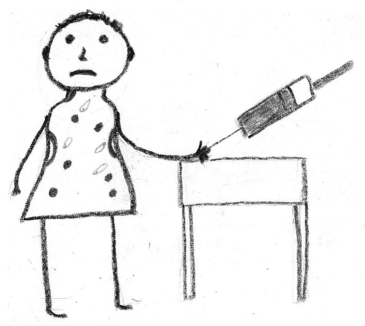

This woman was honest enough to show her conscious despair at the need for chemotherapy, indicated by the sad face and black outline. However, there is a symbolic message from her unconscious telling her to receive the treatment, that it is good for her. The syringe is purple, a spiritual color, and her feet are turned toward the therapy. The image convinced her to try the treatment, and it was successful. Her fears melted away with the tumor.

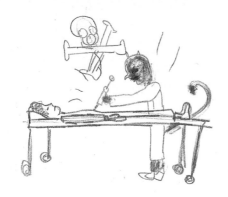

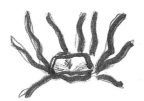

When asked to draw her doctor giving her therapy, Estelle (whose story is told on page 133) drew the Devil giving her poison. She also portrayed her disease as an insect, a negative image considering how hard it is to get rid of insects.

She was sent to my office to help control terrible side effects. The issue was control. She disliked her doctor and didn't want the therapy, but her family urged it upon her. Her recourse was to become so sick they would have to stop treatment.

I told her she had permission to change doctors and stop her therapy—it was her life, not anyone else's. Feeling in control again, she was able to straighten out relationships with her family and doctor, and continue therapy at her desire.

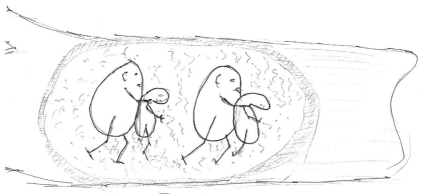

Working lewkocytes: Boy, I'm sure glad these dads are leaving. ~~Hey~~ It'll take us weeks to clean up this mess.

This drawing by Ian is mentioned on page 155. This gentle man taught us all a great deal about healing through love. His white blood cells are carrying his cancer cells away instead of killing them. I feel that images of attacking the disease may work for about 20 percent of patients, but 80 percent need a different approach to heal.

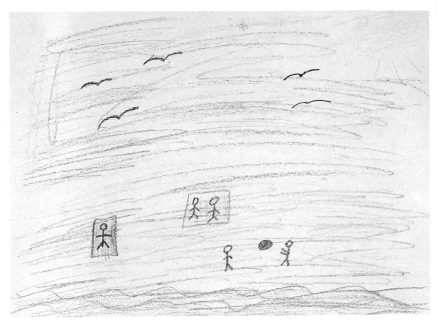

In this drawing of a family on the beach there are five birds and five people, symbolizing and representing the family. Just as three birds are separate, so are three of the people. Three are on beach blankets, but the image really represents their entrapment and inability to help the two who are tossing the ball around or flying alone. The picture dramatized personal problems and conflicts between the parents of a child with cancer.

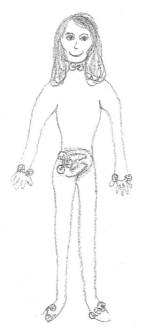

-white blood cells

The whole person represented here has all the assets to help herself change. She has good self-esteem, indicated by the size of the figure on the page, and she stands in a neutral position (hands at her side), with her hands ready to get a grip on things.

I am concerned about the ever-present smile, however. How do we respond when someone asks, "How are you?" or "What's going on in your life?" Symbolically this smile is a performance—like answering "Fine" and "Nothing" to these questions. If we perform we wear ourselves out for the sake of others. Being happy is fine, but performing is self-destructive.

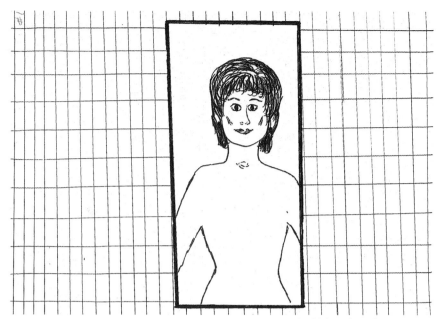

A young lady drew this picture, including every line on the page. She felt boxed in. The entrapment was made up of parental messages: Don't yell. Don't tell anyone your troubles. Don't get a divorce. Don't say no if you want to be liked. Don't, don't, don't—every one another bar in her prison. When she realized what she had displayed, she took her husband and they both went for therapy.

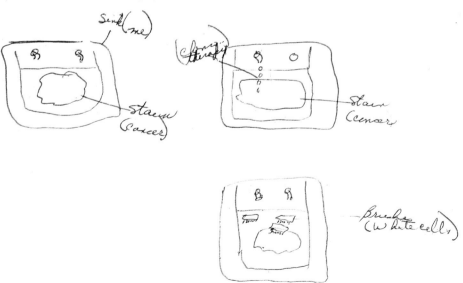

This woman drew herself as a sink because she felt everyone dumped on her. She felt the love she gave was never returned sufficiently. When I said, "If you give up your resentment, you might get well," she said, "No, my resentment and anger keep me alive." Her energy never was utilized for healing, and shortly thereafter she died. Neither physical nor spiritual healing occurred, and her family was left with a lot of painful unfinished business.

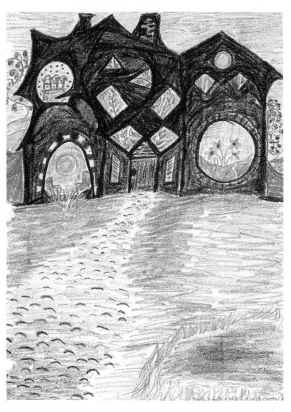

Extensive cancer of the rectum, filling the pelvis, is manifested by a flaming red house, which is symbolically shaped much like the pelvis, with its anal, vaginal, and neurovascular openings.

With psyche and soma being treated, her house changes to a peaceful image, with spirituality coming in and two people (the trees) beginning to help and protect her. The empty windows and lack of a chimney—hot air can't get out, pressure can't be released—speak of a still difficult relationship at home with her husband.

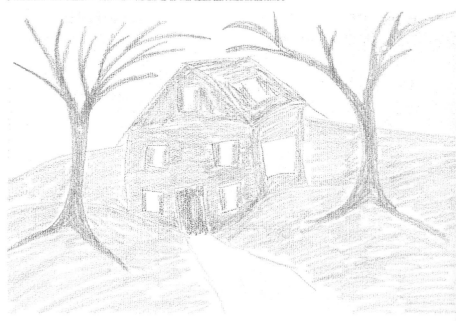

searchers concluded that "blood chemistries offer information only about the current state of the disease, whereas the psychological variables offer future insights" and that "the imagery was found to be the most important in predicting subsequent disease states." By analyzing drawings made by two hundred patients, Achterberg later achieved 95-percent accuracy in predicting who would die within two months and who would be in remission.

The drawing of a young patient named Toby dramatically illustrated the predictive value of images. The young man had had regional enteritis for many years and had become addicted to painkillers. He was so depressed and angry about his condition that he prayed to God every night that he wouldn't wake up the next morning. After two months he decided God probably needed more specific instructions, so he prayed for a brain tumor. In two months he woke up unable to speak, with a brain tumor. Eventually it made him quadriplegic. The experience changed his outlook. Dying in his sleep was okay, but being unable to move or communicate wasn't. Now Toby recalled a visit to me years before. He returned, joined ECaP, and began to see the world with love and express that love to others.

When Toby first came to the group, his tumor was in remission. He drew a tree whose outline looked almost exactly like the brain seen in profile. He pictured black throughout the branches. This let me know that he had a recurring disease, even though his brain scans showed none. I did not depress or frighten him by telling him so. By talking in the group about how he would deal with a recurrence, I was able to help him prepare for what I knew was coming.

In this instance, the tree obviously symbolized the brain. A tree can also stand for many other things, including a person's entire life and development.

After a long battle with his cancer and despite quadriplegia, Toby decided to leave the hospital. At this point when asked how he was Toby responded, "Fine." His answer meant he was at peace and had no fear. To his doctor it meant I was lying to him about his disease. His doctor predicted he would live two weeks and told his mother, "This is no TV program.

It's going to be horrible." His family was able to create a warm, supportive environment, and with love his only therapy he improved to the point where he could move his arms again. His neurologist was courageous enough to visit him at home, and afterward said, "I see what Bernie is talking about."

Toby lived eight more months at home, a time that brought the family closer than ever and helped them share enough love to survive his death. On Memorial Day his breathing became labored, and his mother told him, "Toby, if you want to go it's all right. I'll be okay. We all love you and will miss you, but we'll be all right." He took three breaths and died. The holiday has become a day when he can be with his loved ones, always.

Philosopher Benedetto Croce wrote, "True happiness is to be won by learning to love with such elevation of spirit as to attain the power to stand up to grief. . . . Surpass the old love with an even greater new love." Through his life in those eight months, Toby gave his family the capacity to achieve this kind of love, which helped them all survive and overcome their grief.

The interpretation of drawings is a technique that I'll discuss in a later chapter. Here I merely want to introduce two important symbols—the rainbow and the butterfly. In dreams, mythology, and art, the rainbow is a symbol of hope and a manifestation of our entire emotional spectrum and life. The butterfly is a universal symbol of metamorphosis, a change from ugliness to beauty, from hate to love, and from this life to the next. Children in a Nazi concentration camp scratched butterflies on the walls of their cells. In the excerpt from *Cancer Ward* quoted at the beginning of this book, Aleksandr Solzhenitsyn, himself a survivor of cancer and a concentration camp, brilliantly captured the meaning of these images, out of his unconscious creative awareness.

EXCEPTIONAL DETERMINATION

No matter what their content, the mere fact that a patient is willing to make the drawings shows a basic desire to survive.

It takes courage to do something that will reveal aspects of yourself that you might be more comfortable concealing. Some patients are unwilling to do even this much work, a clear message that they don't want to participate. They say things like "I lost the crayons" or "I can't find the instructions." Others call from out of state to say they'll come to a group meeting tomorrow. I tell them, "Wait. There's some homework first, some reading and some drawings." "Fine," they say. "I'll have it done by tomorrow." It's this type of aggressive patient who has the best chance.

The resolve to do whatever is necessary, including opening up the unconscious, is one of the first requirements for being an exceptional patient. In the next chapter I'll discuss in more detail how to gain the "clear conscience" mentioned by Solzhenitsyn. But no prescription for change will do any good without the courage to accept the challenge—to take control of your life, find your true path, sing your song, and regardless of your age decide what you want to be when you grow up.

Several years ago I received a letter from a remarkable woman named Lois Becker. After hearing of my work, she wrote to share her experience, thanking me for verbalizing what she intuitively knew.

After a terrible year in which her father died of cancer, her husband underwent surgery, her brother was divorced, and her mother and aunt were badly injured in an auto accident, Lois Becker decided to make something good happen by becoming pregnant with her second child. During an examination, her midwife discovered a lump in her right breast and sent her for an immediate biopsy. Her letter continues:

A three-day wait for the results, which I already know in my gut. Three days lying flat on the couch, staring as the television changes programs hour after hour. The phone rings—they'll cut off my breast on Monday. I am thirteen weeks pregnant. I am 33 years old.

They do it. They really meant it. My right side has a 12-inch incision; no lymph glands, no breast. There are 12 more tumors in my glands.

I have three choices: immediate abortion, a caesarean section or induced labor at about 30 weeks, or a full-term delivery. My cancer is hormone-positive, and my body is lousy with hormones. I can't have any of the usual cancer therapy if I keep the baby. Even with an abortion and therapy, my chances are a shattering one in six for five more years of life.

I choose to go for 30 weeks. I don't choose it to save the baby. I choose it to get out of the hospital, so they won't do anything more to me now. They pull two long, sucking tubes out of my side, and I go home. It is January in Minnesota, as frozen as you can get, unless, of course, you are pregnant and have cancer.

When you are a human time-bomb, it is a lot longer than five months from January to May. Each day my baby grows, more of the hormones, so enormously dangerous to me, flood my body. There is little reason to hope that I will complete the pregnancy with no further cancer spread. I am so numb, so angry, so very, very sad that my face freezes into an expressionless mask. I lose the ability to read (previously one of my greatest joys), because my concentration is completely destroyed. I don't expect to see my girl become eight years old on June 30, 1978. I buy all her gifts and wrap them in February. I plan my burial.

But I really was two people, each fighting hard for the upper hand. One heard what the doctors said and reacted as I have just described. But the other shouted obscenities at the hospital whenever her car passed by. This second person decided to fight, even though the first person was after her every day, sometimes every hour, to give up and give in.

Physically, my mastectomy didn't hurt very much. My chest, upper arm, and back were numb, but I healed fast, without complications. But my arm hurt from the beginning, sometimes so badly that I couldn't straighten it for days. Unfortunately it was my right arm, the one I used to strum my guitar. But it really didn't matter, because I wasn't happy enough to sing anymore.

As soon as I left the hospital, I tried to listen to my insides. I wanted my body and mind to tell me how to help them survive. I got some answers, and I tried to follow them even when I was too depressed to move or care. My body said, "Drink orange juice," a curious craving I'd never experienced before. I drank and drank, and it felt right. I put serious thought into what I put into my body. I told my food to make me strong. I told each vitamin, as it slid down my throat, to go to the right places and do the right things, because they were the only cancer pills I had.

My body said, "Move, Lois, and do it fast!" Thirty minutes

after I came home from the hospital I went for a walk. It was hard. I was afraid of falling on my side. I was humped like an old lady. But my legs were strong. I bought a pedometer and walked off miles and miles. When spring came, I walked, ran, walked, and ran, until there was too much baby.

I told my body through exercise that I loved it and wanted it to be healthy. I started yoga again the week I came home. At first I could only move my arm about five inches from my side in any direction, but I stretched and stretched it. I got my three-pound weights out and made my arm muscles and tendons work even though they protested painfully. I got my arm back quickly and have full mobility and strength today. Reach to Recovery says, "Walk your fingers slowly up the door." I say, "Hang on the door, and then do chin-ups if you can."

My mind and body said, "Make love," and they were right. Making love (and other forms of exercise) gave me the only times I was free, the only times I was *me* again, the only times I didn't have cancer.

My mind said, "I need peace. I need some rest every day from the overpowering pressure. Rest me!" I had never meditated, but I went to the library and discovered the forms that worked for me. I practiced. Meditation dropped my tense body out of my waking turmoil into a sweet cradle, deep and dark and refreshingly peaceful. I literally lived for those moments.

Meditation also provided me with a chance to practice medicine without a license. I told my body to be well. I told my immunological system to protect me. I looked at my brain, my bones, my liver, and my lungs every night. I felt them and told them to be free of cancer. I watched my blood flowing strongly. I told the wound to heal quickly and the area around it to be clean. I told my other breast to behave, because it's the only one my husband and I have left. I still tell my body and mind every night, "I reject cancer. I reject cancer."

The doctors poke around, look at my x-rays, let me out into the world again. I make it into spring, into May.

We try an induction the last week in May. It goes on for 10 hours, hurts a lot, and accomplishes nothing. They, the ones not in the bed, want to try again tomorrow. Baby and I want to go home. We go, and I tell myself that three or four more weeks won't kill me! I am happy because, going full term, I can deliver with the midwives. Perhaps the birth, at least, will be beautiful even if the pregnancy was hell.

My college roommate had a baby on June 13, and I guess that I will, too. With amniotic fluid beginning to leak, I go to the hospital to a lovely room with plants and a big double bed. My midwife is good in all ways. The contractions are close and getting stronger, and I begin to lose the fear all women have. I am handling this well. I'm going to enjoy it.

She breaks the bag, and the bed and I are drenched. She says I'm six centimeters, but I watch her face change. I'm pushing the cord out before the baby. I know immediately that he could die—fast. She holds the baby's head off the cord, pushes him up as I push him down, and I now know what the word agony means. As we race to surgery, I hear them say that the baby's pulse rate is 60.

Maybe a C-section was a good idea. They spend another hour looking at my insides. They find nothing but insides, and when my husband tells me, I feel a moment of great relief.

The baby is an 8-pound, 1/2-ounce, 21-inch baby boy named Nathan Scott. He is very cute, with brown hair, long dark eyelashes—and a large ventricular septal defect, known among the lucky uninitiated as a heart murmur or hole-in-the-heart. It is congenital. It is serious. It will probably need surgery. It might kill him. And, worst of all for me, it means constant trips to a hospital I hate, trips that leave me exhausted and depressed for days. It means letting my baby be cut up, just like me, for his own good.

Nathan is in congestive heart failure for the first six months of his life. He takes digitalis twice a day. He sweats when he eats. His little bony chest rises and falls much too fast, and his liver and heart are enlarged. He goes into the hospital for awhile. I stay with him, and it causes me nearly to break. His original 50-percent chance of closure drops to 25 percent.

But then, sometime in his seventh month, he begins to improve. (I like to think it was during one of those moments when I was whispering in his little ear, "Nathan, you are *going* to get well!")

The doctors are surprised. The EKGs improve. He gains weight. His breathing slows and the liquid swelling leaves his liver.

In May 1979 Nate has his first normal EKG, a better event than a first birthday. The muscle has closed around the hole.

Nathan pulls himself up on his feet and stands tall, and I begin to believe in his existence.

When my tummy flattened out, I had a big surprise. I really *didn't* have a breast on the right side. Now was the time when most new mothers love to put on their old clothes, or buy new ones, or dream of two-piece bathing suits. My tent clothes had protected me for six months. Now I had to confront my true feelings about my body, another struggle to add to all the rest.

To describe how I felt as depression is mild. But I kept pushing myself to continue the positive elements in my life. For seven months I didn't lose my baby fat, but when Nathan began to improve, I experienced a new wave of determination.

I lost 20 pounds. I continued to meditate and to swallow all my vitamins. Three months after the birth I rejoined my exercise group. Now I didn't have to walk; I could run. And I run so well I'm planning to enter some races. My exercise program consists of yoga, running, and biking. I do them every day. I have to. I believe they are helping me survive.

My figure is back, with clothes on anyway. I'm even beginning to think I don't look too grotesque with them off. My C-section scar didn't do much to help my self-image, but my husband is blind when he looks at my scars, and I am learning to see through his eyes.

I began to try to learn how to put *myself* first. No one helped me with this. No one suggested I even had a chance. The doctors totally depressed me with their statistics. Well meaning acquaintances practically destroyed me with their pity. But in spite of other people, what *I* did worked, and each day of continued good health makes me more confident of "mind over matter."

I think of cancer every day, but I also think of how strong my body is, how good it feels most of the time. I still talk to my insides. I have a feeling of integration of body, mind and, probably, spirit, which I have never before experienced. Cancer introduced me to myself, and I like who I met.

After six years in a remission of her own doing, Lois died, but the quality of her life during that time was something her doctors never predicted. Cancer generally seems to appear in response to loss, such as the tragedies that occurred in Lois's family during the year before her tumor developed. I believe that, if a person avoids emotional growth at this time, the impulse behind it becomes misdirected into malignant physical growth. As Jungian therapist Russell A. Lockhart wrote:

> The phenomenology of cancer is full of images of guilt and retribution and promises to oneself and others that, should there be recovery, sacrifices will be made, there will be a change of ways, life will be lived properly. The psychology of such unwilling sacrifice is quite different from that of the willing sacrifice.
>
> There are moments and seasons in one's life when genuine sacrifice of the most valued thing is essential for further growth. If this sacrifice is not made willingly, that is, consciously and with full conscious suffering of the loss, the sacrifice will occur unconsciously. One then will not sacrifice to growth, but be sacrificed to growth gone wrong.

By the same token, subsequent psychological and spiritual development is capable of reversing the disease process. It's as though cancer's energy is channeled into self-discovery, and the tumor is attacked by the immune system. The tumor is now an estranged and unnecessary part. It's almost as though the individual is reborn and rejects the old self, and its disease, thereby becoming able to identify the tumor as something distinct and separate from the new self. The change is strikingly similar to discoveries in recent work with multiple-personality patients: One personality may be diabetic, while the other is not. Allergies and drug sensitivities may be present in one personality but not in others. If one personality burns the body with a cigarette, the mark may disappear when the other personality is in control and reappear when the first personality reappears. Similarly, when a patient with a physical illness makes a thorough and positive personality change, the body's defenses may now eliminate the disease, which is not part of the new self.

II

EMBODYING
THE
MIND

5

*The world is not divine play, it is divine fate. That
there are world, man, the human person, you and I,
has divine meaning.
Creation—happens to us, burns into us, changes
us, we tremble and swoon, we submit. Creation—we
participate in it, we encounter the creator, offer
ourselves to Him, helpers and companions.*

—MARTIN BUBER

Beginning the Journey

A patient's effort to take responsibility and participate in medical choices must begin while he or she is still fighting the shock of the diagnosis and trying to mobilize the will to live. As discussed in Chapter 2, it is the doctor's duty to try immediately to forge a bond of trust by learning and accepting the patient's beliefs, conscious and unconscious. The quickest way to develop patients' trust and independence is simply to be human, to share their pain, and avoid playing the role of a mechanic-lifesaver. But, because so many doctors are caught up in that role, patients often must help change them. Toward this end, I advise patients to insist on the following Patient's Bill of Rights, in the form of an open letter to physicians:

Dear Doctor:

Please don't conceal the diagnosis. We both know I came to you to learn if I have cancer or some other serious disease. If I know what I have, I know what I am fighting, and there is less to fear. If you hide the name and the facts, you deprive me of the chance to help myself. When you are questioning whether I should be told, I already know. You may feel better if you don't tell me, but your deception hurts me.

Do not tell me how long I have to live! I alone can decide how long I will live. It is my desires, my goals, my values, my strengths, and my will to live that will make the decision.

Teach me and my family about how and why my illness happened to me. Help me and my family to live *now*. Tell me about nutrition and my body's needs. Tell me how to handle the knowledge and how my mind and body can work together. Healing comes from within, but I want to combine my strength with yours. If you and I are a team, I will live a longer and better life.

Doctor, don't let your negative beliefs, your fears, and your prejudices affect my health. Don't stand in the way of my getting well and exceeding your expectations. Give me the chance to be the exception to your statistics.

Teach me about your beliefs and therapies and help me to incorporate them into mine. However, remember that my beliefs are the most important. What I don't believe in won't help me.

You must learn what my disease means to me—death, pain, or fear of the unknown. If my belief system accepts alternative therapy and not recognized therapy, do not desert me. Please try to convert my beliefs, and be patient and await my conversion. It may come at a time when I am desperately ill and in great need of your therapy.

Doctor, teach me and my family to live with my problem when I am not with you. Take time for our questions and give us your attention when we need it. It is important that I feel free to talk with you and question you. I will live a longer and more meaningful life if you and I can develop a significant relationship. I need you in my life to achieve my new goals.

HELPING PATIENTS MAKE CHOICES

I always try to get patients to see standard medical treatments—such as radiation, chemotherapy, and surgery—as energy that can heal them. They buy time during which I can help the patient find the will to live, change, and heal. Many of the disagreements over the worth of alternate therapies arise because some people heal themselves no matter what external aids they choose, as long as they have hope and some control over the therapy. I support them as long as a patient has chosen them with a positive conviction, not out of fear. When a patient says, "I'm scared to death of surgery" and therefore chooses something else, I can't support that choice.

Affirmation aids the body, fear is destructive. Treatment chosen out of fear is unlikely to be helpful.

I try to get patients to understand that the *body* heals, not the therapy. All healing is scientific. At a recent conference, someone told me he knew someone on a macrobiotic diet, someone else on a diet exactly the opposite, and a third person on chemotherapy and radiation. All three got well, and this person couldn't understand how the body could accomplish this or how the treatments made any sense. But the body can utilize any form of energy for healing—even Krebiozen or plain water—as long as the patient believes in it.

Let's say I recommended eating three peanut butter sandwiches a day to cure cancer. Some people would get well and claim it was the peanut butter that did it. Then even more people would have hope, eat peanut butter, and get better, too. But we know it's not the peanut butter. It's their hope and the changes they produce in their lives while they're on the new therapy.

The most important thing is to pick a therapy you believe in and proceed with a positive attitude. Each person must chart his own course. One may want a comprehensive nutritional supplement program, while another thinks taking dozens of pills a day is too much of a nuisance, and it becomes counterproductive. Some can just "leave their troubles to God" and be healed. Others need what I call the "football coach" method, in which the patient plans every detail. I thought of the phrase while working with Eileen, a patient who saw a hypnotherapist regularly, picked the date for surgery herself, and hired private-duty nurses. She made sure she was in control of the situation and ready for every eventuality. She is alive and well today, having recently celebrated a year cancer-free anniversary with a big party at her house. Her message to others with cancer is, "Here's the information. Go and *do it.*"

Since cancer patients typically feel little control over their lives, to the point where their own cells are in revolt, the mere fact of making a choice can itself be a turning point. For Herbert Howe that moment came when he decided to stop chemotherapy because it was making him too sick. His oncologist told him he was crazy and would soon die. That angered

Howe so much that he wanted to hit his oncologist. Instead he went out and started jogging. Since then, he has practically made a career out of exercise—running, rowing, climbing mountains, and in general putting all his energy into life and living. Seven years later he is free of disease.

Training patients in meditation is one of the best ways to help them past their fear to choices based on their own beliefs. This was dramatically borne out by the experience of Bruce, a family therapist who took up meditation after hearing one of my talks. Bruce had become addicted to opiates and alcohol after using them for the pain of recovery from a skiing accident. He developed severe liver disease and a portacaval shunt was recommended, to allow the blood to bypass the diseased liver. While meditating, he heard an inner voice saying, "You have to turn the tide." The voice later gave him a four-point program:

1. A week of intravenous vitamin C.
2. Daily meditation.
3. Consultation with a nutritionist.
4. Use of a computer.

At this time Bruce knew nothing about the value of intravenous vitamin C in such conditions, but he found someone to administer it to him anyway. The last bit of advice was puzzling until a few days later, when he read a newspaper article about programming a computer to deliver subliminal messages. Having access to a computer, Bruce created an image of a spiritual figure protecting and healing him, and programmed the machine to flash this image repeatedly on the video screen. Other people have shown that subliminal images of white cells eating cancer cells also help patients get better. In a few months Bruce's liver tests were normal, he conquered his other problems, and required no surgery.

Group discussion is also immensely helpful in convincing patients that they *can* choose a course that feels right to them. In ECaP we have had people on laetrile, vitamin C, strict dietary regimens, standard therapy only, and some on no medical therapy at all. At first I was worried that people would argue over who was doing the right thing. Instead, they all share the belief that they will get well. They waste no energy on deciding whose therapy is better. The diversity opens people's minds to other allies in the struggle and helps them see that there's no single answer, that in a sense any path can be the right one. The group is a family but more open than most families. It's an environment where it's safe to say and feel anything, where those further along in their psychological development become "therapists" to help the newcomers find meaning in their lives, no matter what treatment they've chosen.

In general I feel it's best for patients to focus their energy on one or two approaches they believe in most strongly. However, many actions—such as nutritional supplementation, exercise, and meditation—are valuable aids to any treatment and therefore are important parts of the ECaP program.

When a patient wants to fly to Mexico and take laetrile, I ask, "Why are you going? What are your beliefs? What are your fears?" If the response is, "Gee, it costs a lot of money. Should I go?" I say, "No, not if you're questioning it." But if the person has a confirmed belief in laetrile, I may support the trip, even though I may say, "I wouldn't do that if I had what you have." But I always tell the patient, "I'm here as another option if this doesn't work out for you."

MINIMIZING SIDE EFFECTS

I don't try to browbeat people into receiving radiation or chemotherapy if they think these are toxic, because they'll prove themselves right. They'll have every possible side effect and then say, "Look what this has done to me. I shouldn't have listened to you." Or they'll resist more directly by simply flushing their medicine down the toilet. One ECaP member's oncologist gave her a certain drug regimen with instructions to take one pill each day for a week, but without telling her there were only five pills in the package. She later called her oncologist to say that she was vomiting and didn't have enough pills for the full seven days. He told her, "We'll adjust the dose, but in two years you're the first patient who has ever called to complain about not having enough pills." Apparently many of the others had just thrown them away when they started vomiting. Dr. Alexandra Levine found that 60 percent of patients in a survey she conducted had no trace of medication in their blood samples. Yet chemotherapy statistics are based on the assumption that all patients take their drugs. Many oncologists now insist that patients take the pills under supervision, but an open, trusting relationship would be better.

In my opinion, about three-fourths of the side effects of radiation and chemotherapy result from patients' negative beliefs, fostered by a destructive kind of hypnosis on the part of the physician. Most doctors say something like "All these bad things can happen to you, and if you're lucky something good might happen." No good hypnotherapist would ever write a protocol like those usually given to cancer patients. All the things that are going to go wrong are listed first, so everybody is put into a "no" mode. By the time you get to the bottom of the page, where it suggests that good things may happen, you continue to say, "No, no, no."

Nobody's going to sue a doctor for accenting the positive, and the physician doesn't have to make any guarantees. All that's necessary is to change the emphasis: "A lot of good things can happen because of this treatment. It is possible the following adverse effects may occur, but I don't expect them." That way, patients will be saying, "Yes, yes, yes," and then at the bottom of the page they'll be convinced they're unlikely to have any of the following side effects. Patients should also be reminded that normal cells can recover from the strong medicines better than weak, sensitive cancer cells.

The experience of one of our group members, a physician named Martin, illustrates this point perfectly. Before he went for chemotherapy, we talked about the power of expectation in determining one's reactions. Martin's oncologist's nurse told him to take his antinausea pill at 8 P.M., the chemotherapy pills at 9 P.M., and another antinausea pill at 10 P.M. Then the patient was directed to spread newspapers across his bedroom rug in case he couldn't make it to the bathroom in time, and have a bucket near the bed with some water in it so the vomit wouldn't stick to the pail. The instructions so unnerved him that it took him an extra two hours to start taking the pills. Then, remembering our talk, Martin kept reminding himself to think of the good things that could happen instead of the bad. Finally he took all the medication, fell asleep, and woke up the next morning without any problems. He said, "If we had not talked I couldn't have done it."

Negative programming is one reason why a fourth of all chemotherapy patients start throwing up *before* they get to their next treatment. In England a group of men were given saline and told it was chemotherapy, 30 percent had their hair fall out. Behavioral scientists have shown that the techniques used to conquer phobias can eliminate this anticipatory nausea, but they are usually not needed when chemotherapy is given in a sharing doctor-patient relationship, along with imagery training and attention to the patient's emotional problems. Patients can also take a portable tape recorder to bring music or positive messages with them to the doctor's office, creating a controlled environment to help themselves through the therapy. A woman named Estelle was sent to me because of the incredible side effects she was having. When I asked her to draw her treatment, she drew the devil giving her poison. She had been hiding the way she really felt about her doctor and treatment, but we were able to clarify the problem, restore control to her, not the family, and alter her relationship with her doctor, allowing her to go back to treatment.

When I can see patients before therapy and help them with the decision, they have far fewer problems with treatment than other patients. Then marijuana or anti-emetic drugs are unnecessary. Marie, one of our patients, was told that she would have nausea. She said she wouldn't but the doctor and staff insisted she take some Compazine home with her. She said, "I went home, and about an hour or two later I belched and thought, 'Oops, it's probably going to start.'" So she went to the drawer, took out a pill, swallowed it, and immediately felt better. A few hours later she belched again and yelled to her daughter, "Would you please get me my Compazine pill from the dresser?"

After about fifteen minutes, her daughter said, "Mom, I

can't find any Compazine pills here. There's Coumadin." Marie had seen a pill with a large C on it, presumed it was a Compazine, swallowed it, and immediately felt well anyway. Coumadin is an anticoagulant but worked for Marie as a wonderful placebo. Then she realized she'd been doing a mind job on herself. They'd been talking her into nausea, but she didn't need either the side effect or the pill.

I remember a woman named Lillian, who at first couldn't even sit in our group's circle. "I'm not used to sharing these kinds of things with people," she said. Eventually she not only joined the circle but went on TV with me and several other patients. One of Lillian's biggest problems had been chemotherapy side effects. She got sick on the way to the doctor and used marijuana to partially counteract the nausea. After our counseling, she talked over the problem with her doctor. Then one day in the group she asked, "Who knows when I received my chemotherapy?" No one did. "I got it forty-five minutes ago," she exulted, "and here I am feeling fine."

Another patient, Maxine, came to me after a recurrence of breast cancer. After excising a nodule in her armpit, I suggested radiation and chemotherapy. Maxine ran a health-food store and had not taken a pill in seventeen years, so she didn't think she could accept my suggestion. She'd heard of all the side effects and all her friends told her what a terrible time she would have.

I explained that these treatments can help, with tolerable or nonexistent side effects, if one believes in them and sees treatment as energy. I told her about a similar patient who, when her oncologist started to outline all the adverse reactions, interrupted, "Oh, I won't have any. You forget who my surgeon is." One week of constipation was the sum total of her chemotherapy side effects, and during treatment she worked her normal schedule as a teacher.

I tried to get Maxine to think of both forms of therapy as energy that the body could use to heal itself. She said she could visualize x-ray treatment that way, and she had an excellent response to it. Later she came to see chemotherapy as energy, too, with further positive results. She continued to run her store and take care of her children. Her dreams during therapy reflected her conflict. She dreamed of a gardener and cleaning woman, who worked with natural materials but also used chemical fertilizers and caustic cleaning agents. By confronting her fears in discussion, however, she was able to accept the therapy and let it work for her. All her friends warned her about the poisons she was using, but her improving health surprised them and changed their beliefs.

Sometimes a surprisingly simple act can change the conditioning. One ECaP member always used to throw up immediately after her chemotherapy. Her husband would always have a bag ready for her to throw up in as she got into the car. But one day she opened the bag and found a dozen roses. She never threw up after chemotherapy again.

EFFECTIVE BELIEFS

Beliefs shape the power of the treatment as well as the seriousness of its side effects. Radiation can be a killer ray or a golden beam of healing energy. Since chemotherapy attacks primarily cells with a fast metabolic rate, such as those in tumors and hair follicles, loss of hair can and should be interpreted as evidence that the medicine is working. For those who don't want to lose their hair an ice cap or similar visualization technique can work. They have to remember that they will not have this sign as a therapeutic effect. One nurse believed so strongly in her treatments that she called herself a chemotherapy junkie. Greta, another ECaP member, imagined her chemotherapy as "scrubbing bubbles" from a TV commercial for bathroom cleanser. She told her doctor he didn't need to describe every possible side effect, that she would talk with him if anything came up, but he didn't have to program her in a negative way. She never had any significant adverse reactions.

Greta later said, "I believe cancer is the best thing that ever happened to me. If I can help someone else know how they can fight cancer, it's all worthwhile. I'm sure that's why I got cancer." Patients who say this or similar things are those whose lives have been so filled with pain that the redirection caused by the illness is profoundly important, bringing new meaning and love into their lives. It doesn't mean they wouldn't get rid of the disease in a minute if they could, but they wouldn't give up the changes it brought. The desire to learn from this experience and help others makes any treatment more bearable. As Dr. Kenneth Cohn wrote after his recovery from lymphoma, "The opportunity for personal growth during chemotherapy can and should be conveyed to patients, because the heightened self-esteem which results from that growth will increase patients' stamina . . . and diminish the likelihood of their discontinuing therapy prematurely."

No matter what method is chosen to restore physical health, it's essential to plan it so that it doesn't impair mental health. Chemotherapy regimens, for example, can be adjusted to fit the other important things in a person's life. A young man named Denny was referred to me by his oncologist because of terrible side effects to chemotherapy. When he came to my office, Denny said, "Don't say 'it.' "

I asked, "What's 'it'?"

He said, "You know what 'it' is."

"Cancer?" I asked.

"Yes," he said, and went to the sink and threw up. He told me, "I'm given my medication on Friday night and Saturday so I'll be sick on the weekend and then be able to go back to college on Monday. But I can't date and I can't participate in sports."

I asked him why he didn't have his treatment on Monday. He said, "My oncologist and my mother think this is the best program, and it's part of the protocol."

I told him, "Well, it's your life, but if I were you I'd skip a weekend or perhaps have it on Monday, so you can enjoy your life."

Next week on Friday I got a phone call asking if I knew where Denny was. A few hours later I got a phone call from Montreal. He'd driven the family jalopy to Montreal to see his girlfriend. He returned on Monday for chemotherapy, and had no side effects. He was able to complete his course of therapy with no further problems, and he is well today.

On the next Thursday Denny's mother came to an ECaP meeting. At first I thought she was going to wallop me with her pocketbook, but she said, "No, I knew you were right." When I asked her why, she said, "Well, he drove all the way to Montreal and back in the family jalopy. I wouldn't have gone around the corner in that car. On Monday when he got back, I *did* go around the corner, and it broke down. I knew he had spiritual guidance!"

ECaP's main goal is to foster this kind of autonomy and awareness in patients and their loved ones by helping them achieve the peace of mind that enables them to deal with life's issues. We've come to believe that the resolution of conflicts, the realization of the authentic self, spiritual awareness, and love release incredible energy that promotes the biochemistry of healing.

We had a physician named Herb who came to our group. He said he meditated every night while he walked the dog. One night, while walking down the street, he heard God say to him, "You are Jesus."

Herb said, "I'm Jewish."

God said, "I know that. So was Jesus."

Herb thought, "I guess God is telling me to heal myself by the laying on of hands." He started patting himself all over as he stood out there in the street.

When he came to the group and told this story, I asked him, "Did it ever occur to you that God was saying, 'You need to become loving and spiritual'? Being a physician, you reacted in a mechanical way and did something mechanical, like patting yourself all over, but the message is 'Change and be spiritual.'"

In ECaP we promote these changes in weekly two-hour group meetings. ECaP is a nonprofit corporation. We charge a modest fee to defray costs, but anyone who cannot afford it is admitted free. Personally, I feel this is a form of therapy that no one should consider as his sole source of income. I spend large amounts of time with patients, and I never want them to be thinking, "How much will this cost me?"

No physician's referral is needed, and no one is ever turned away. The only admission requirements are that people do the drawings and fill out the admission form with the four questions and request for historical information. Each member begins by doing a drawing of himself, his disease, his white blood cells, and his treatment. We then discuss these drawings in at least one individual session before the patient joins one of the groups. We maintain a lending library to encourage members to become as well informed as possible. We supply members with an assortment of self-help educational materials.

In our group sessions we discuss every aspect of our lives —treatment goals and options, nutrition, exercise, the psychological origins of disease, management of pain and fear, and techniques of stress reduction. We help patients set goals for their lives, find occasions for play and laughter, deal with sexual problems, and develop an emotional support system among friends and family. Most of all, we seek to help them rise to what for most is the supreme challenge of their lives, by developing *and enjoying* their unique personalities to the fullest. In many ways we try to accomplish what Alcoholics Anonymous tries to do for alcoholics—changes in lifestyle, acceptance of responsibility, spiritual awareness, sharing. Like AA, we provide an "instant family," which is nonjudgmental. In general, we discuss why we're alive and what we're here for. Each session closes with a period of meditation and guided imagery, and we help patients adapt these techniques for their daily use. The ECaP family is often more loving and supportive than the biological one.

An oncologist once asked me, "Since you're not trained in psychotherapy, how do you know you won't do these patients harm?" I replied, "I love them. I may not help, but I'm sure I won't hurt them." ECaP can be supplemented by further psychotherapy, but a patient facing a life-threatening illness may not have the luxury of in-depth analysis. Reliving self-destructive tendencies is not a live message. We need to utilize a therapeutic approach that makes life joyful. I tell patients "Deal with your emotions and live as if you were going to die tomorrow. Later, if you still need to, you may have the time to look back and discover why you are who you are."

In ECaP's seven years, we have had only two letters questioning what we were doing, and both came from psychiatrists who seemed worried about losing control over their patients. One protested our giving his patient a book, and the other condemned our helping a patient who had stopped his anti-depressant medication. I have no qualms about recommending the same approach to other doctors, no matter what their training. Caring is the key. Studies have shown that when you put a janitor in a psychiatrist's office, the patients get better—as long as the janitor is empathetic.

The remainder of this chapter concerns the "externals" of the program—methods for changing *what you do*. In the following chapters we will explore the "internals"—ways to change *who you are*. Please keep in mind that most of the discussion concerns cancer because, as a surgeon, I see many cancer patients. However, I believe that the same practices improve the prospects in all diseases, and in ECaP we have seen positive results with diabetes, scleroderma, multiple sclerosis, arthritis, neurologic disorders, obesity, asthma, AIDS, cancer. One patient came because of cancer but was more concerned with his asthma. After a few months of work on lifestyle changes, meditation, and imagery, he needed no cortisone and almost no other medication. That was when he became convinced that he was on the right track, because in his family asthma and emphysema, not cancer, have always been the killers. As oncologist Sam Bobrow said in reply to a Boston *Globe* reporter who asked how my patients do, "It's not clear to me that patients live longer with Bernie, but they feel better while they're living, and that's what's important." But I say, "Show me a patient who enjoys living and I'll show you someone who is going to live longer."

NUTRITION

Good nutrition is an essential part of any treatment program, but I don't believe in prescribing a strict regimen for all patients. I give patients dietary guidelines and make vitamin supplements available from my office, but I think it's more important to get people to love themselves and listen to their bodies. If people don't care about themselves, they won't follow my advice to exercise, eat right, and not smoke. Information on sensible nutrition is available from many sources, and I urge people to seek it out and become expert. Many patients have lost contact with their physical selves, just as people sitting in a room with a clock grow so used to its ticking that they no longer hear it. I try to help patients reestablish communication between mind and body. Then they not only eat the right foods, but they also can use their mental powers for healing.

In general, I recommend the type of diet advocated by the late health researcher Nathan Pritikin—which is the type eaten in countries where people regularly live to be a hundred —or one based on the following dietary guidelines prepared by the American Institute for Cancer Research and endorsed by the National Academy of Sciences:

1. Reduce the intake of dietary fat—both saturated and unsaturated—to a maximum level of 30 percent of total calories. This can be done by limiting the use of meat, trimming away its excess fat, avoiding fried foods, and cutting down on butter, cream, salad dressings, and so forth.
2. Increase the consumption of fresh fruits, vegetables, and whole-grain cereals. This automatically increases one's intake of the following five nutrients known to have a protective effect against cancer: beta carotene (a vegetable precursor of vitamin A), vitamin C, vitamin E, selenium, and dietary fiber.
3. Consume salt-cured and charcoal-broiled foods only in moderation (or not at all).
4. Drink alcoholic beverages only in moderation (or not at all).

In addition, the Pritikin-type regimen eliminates from the diet:

1. Nearly all salt except that found in food itself.
2. All stimulants like coffee and tea.

3. All refined sugar and flour.
4. Hydrogenated fats.
5. Pepper and other hot spices.
6. Foods containing artificial additives or preservatives.

This last piece of advice covers nitrite-cured meats such as hot dogs, and may be broadened to include all commercial meats from animals fed hormones, antibiotics, and other feed additives.

Some former cancer patients attribute their recovery to strict dietary regimens. For example, Dr. Anthony Sattilaro, president of Methodist Hospital in Philadelphia, credits his conquest of advanced prostatic cancer, with bone metastases, to macrobiotics, a unified approach to life that emphasizes not only diet but also thoughts and lifestyle. His account of the experience in *Recalled by Life*, written with Tom Monte, includes a wonderful example of the way a teacher often appears as if by magic just when the need is greatest. Sattilaro's father had just died of cancer and, overwhelmed with the knowledge that he was dying too, the son did something he never did before—on the way back from the funeral he picked up two hitchhikers. One of them happened to be a macrobiotic chef, who told the doctor he didn't necessarily have to die and started him on the road to recovery.

I do believe in synchronicity, or meaningful coincidence. However, I don't recommend picking up hitchhikers, and I don't force vegetarianism on patients. I think one's mental and spiritual outlook is more important to health than any particular diet, although vegetarians with cancer do have better survival statistics. Vegetarian Seventh Day Adventists have a lower incidence of colonic and rectal cancer than the rest of the American population, but Utah Mormons have even less, despite a per-capita beef consumption slightly *higher* than the U.S. average.

I remember a cancer patient named Charlie, who loved salami and hot dogs. Despite his illness, he would ask his wife to buy these processed meats. She would bring them home, but, feeling they were wrong for him, put them in the garbage disposal, and the two of them would yell at each other. When Charlie asked me what was correct, I told him I thought feeling good was more important. The sermons and "Don't die" messages from his family were not helping, only creating conflicts. I feel it's important to eat sensibly but just as important to make sure that meals are a pleasure, not a joyless burden. So I told Charlie, "If I had extensive cancer that had spread to my liver, nobody would stop me from eating a hot dog if I wanted to eat one. However, when you come to the point where you enjoy living and feel these foods are inappropriate for you, you will stop eating them."

EXERCISE

Our bodies were designed to move, and they can't stay healthy if we spend all our time sitting or lying down. People who exercise regularly have fewer illnesses than sedentary persons. In the hospital, those who get up and walk as soon as possible are the ones who recover most quickly from surgery.

Vigorous exercise benefits the body both directly and indirectly. It stimulates the immune system and enables us to cope with stress. Many experiments have shown that, when animals are stressed and not allowed physical activity, their bodies degenerate. When given the same stresses and the freedom to exercise, however, they remain healthy. Back in the 1930s, two researchers were able to vary the incidence of tumors in a strain of cancer-prone mice from 16 to 88 percent merely by raising some on calorie-restricted diets and plentiful exercise, while giving others unlimited food and little opportunity for physical activity. In 1960, another group of scientists found that an extract of exercised muscle, when injected into mice with cancer, slowed the growth of tumors and sometimes eliminated them entirely. An extract of nonexercised muscle had no effect.

The psychological benefits are just as important. Just the act of setting aside a regular time for this fundamental and rewarding activity gives a greater sense of self-esteem and control over one's life. Moreover, all forms of exercise help you "hear" your body and its needs, while shutting out other concerns. Exercise, especially running, walking, swimming, and other repetitive types, offers a chance to meditate, because we don't have to think about what we're doing. This will benefit anyone, as long as the exercise doesn't become a way to "run away" from problems or an excuse to stay away from one's family. Exercise has been successfully used to treat depression, and for the same reasons it is a potent weapon against physical afflictions.

The type and amount can only be worked out on an individual basis. I recommend one half hour to one hour daily or every other day, according to what is comfortable for the individual. Just remember that a sick body demands a slower pace than a healthy one. Warning signals of pain or excessive fatigue must be heeded, but they're signs to ease up, not to stop entirely. The most important thing is that if exercise becomes work it defeats its purpose. Instead of a time of communication between mind and body, it becomes just one more stress. It's up to each person to choose activities that he or she enjoys and to exercise only to the point of relaxation, pleasant tiredness, and a little perspiration. When you can't exercise you can visualize yourself exercising and this stimulates your body also. I utilize this technique on long drives.

PLAY AND LAUGHTER

A college professor was lying helpless on the operating table just before surgery, when one of the nurses mentioned that she was one of his former students. "I hope I passed you," he quipped. Laughter, which Sir William Osler called "the music of life," makes the unbearable bearable, and a patient with a well-developed sense of humor has a better chance of recovery than a stolid individual who seldom laughs.

I remember Joselle, an ECaP member with an exceptional sense of humor. Though quite a hefty woman, she would come to meetings wearing a tight shirt, shorts, high socks, and an outlandish hat—all as sort of a performance to give the others a laugh. One day she said that her chest x-ray showed the cancer was going away. I said, "I know why." Everyone leaned forward, waiting for some erudite explanation. "It's because no self-respecting cancer would appear in an outfit like that." People continue to see humor if they retain a childlike spirit—that is, a sense of innocence and play—and I know Joselle's sense of humor contributed to her progress. As long as people are alive, things can still be funny, and we can help them laugh.

There are sound scientific reasons why we call robust, unrestrained laughter "hearty." It produces complete, relaxed action of the diaphragm, exercising the lungs, increasing the blood's oxygen level, and gently toning the entire cardiovascular system. Norman Cousins termed it "internal jogging," and others have likened it to a deep massage. A story or situation that we anticipate will be funny creates a rising level of tension reflected in pulse, skin temperature, and blood pressure. This tension is suddenly released in muscular contractions with the punch line. All the muscles of the chest, abdomen, and face get a little workout, and if the joke is a real knee slapper, even the arms and legs reap the benefits. After the laughter, all the muscles are relaxed, including the heart—the pulse rate and blood pressure temporarily decline. Physiologists have found that muscle relaxation and anxiety cannot exist together, and the relaxation response after a good laugh has been measured as lasting as long as forty-five minutes.

According to some scientific studies, laughter also increases the production of a class of brain chemicals called catecholamines. These include the compounds that, in some circumstances, stimulate the fight-or-flight response, which may inhibit healing. However, increased amounts of some of these compounds in the blood can also reduce inflammation by activating a different part of the immune system. In addition, they increase the production of endorphins, the body's natural opiates. It appears that these are two of the things that happen during laughter. Thus humor may relieve pain directly, by physiological means, as well as by diverting our attention and helping us relax. Norman Cousins, when watching *Candid*

Camera and Marx brothers tapes while fighting ankylosing spondylitis, found that ten minutes of hearty laughter gave him two hours of pain-free sleep. Since nearly every hospital room has a TV set, I hope someday we have a "healing channel" that includes plenty of comedy, as well as music, meditation, and healing imagery.

Humor's most important psychological function is to jolt us out of our habitual frame of mind and promote new perspectives. Psychologists have long noted that one of the best measures of mental health is the ability to laugh at oneself in a gently mocking way—like the dear old schoolteacher, a colostomy patient of mine several years ago, who named her two stomas Harry and Larry. When she would call me and say Harry was acting up again, her lightheartedness helped both of us deal with the situation.

Julie, a young lady who came to ECaP because of blindness resulting from diabetes, showed us all how laughter makes life better. Once, when out to dinner at a restaurant her family and friends sat her down in a chair, and she, presuming the table was in front of her, inched her chair forward. She kept inching and inching, and ended up across the room. Everyone was silent, not knowing how to respond. Finally, she bumped into another table, where the people asked, "Would you like to join us?" As soon as she realized what had happened, she started laughing, and the whole restaurant exploded in laughter.

One day Julie was walking with her boyfriend, who kept telling her, "Be careful. Step down. Step up." He was so concerned about her that *he* fell off the curb. So she handed him her cane and said, "Here, you need this more than I do." Julie has since regained her sight—truly a healing miracle—and no longer fears blindness. Her statement to me was, "Blindness taught me to see, and death taught me to live." She is now one of our co-therapists.

Exercise, laughter, and play are closely related. All three need to be approached in much the same spirit, all three produce similar effects on body and mind. Humor is an essential part of our group experiences in ECaP. We may cry, but we also laugh. We work with people to help them release the child within, for we find that rigid persons who can't let themselves play are the ones who have the hardest time healing or changing their lives to deal with illness. There are individuals who must have play assigned to them in order not to feel guilty playing.

When someone draws his emotions as a little black box or a tight red circle, it's easy to see how restricted the expression of feeling can be. The same is true of positive feelings. As adults, many people must struggle to overcome a lifetime of conditioning and destructive messages, such as, "Be brave," "Be perfect," "Hurry up," "Try harder," "Be strong," and "Please me." Consequently, many people have to "work" at playing. Carl Simonton was such a person. He assigned himself a regular period of play and took up juggling to let his inner child out. In this way he was able to become something he was not conditioned to be. He worked at playing.

We must learn to give fun a high priority in life. Like all other positive change, this also develops from the essential first step—learning to love ourselves. Each of us must take the time to find humorous books or movies, play the games we enjoy, tell jokes to friends, doodle, or have fun with coloring books, whatever the choice is of the child inside you. Not only does play make you feel good; it's also a disinhibitor that opens the door to creativity, an essential element of the inner changes we'll be talking about in Chapter 8. Choose to love and make others happy, and your life will change, because you will find happiness and love in the process. The first step towards inner peace is to decide to give love not receive it.

6

Focusing the Mind for Healing

Basic techniques for contacting the unconscious mind and harnessing its powers have been a standard part of people's education in many cultures, especially in the East and in preindustrial, tribal societies. In the West, such methods have been almost totally neglected in favor of logical processes based on the three Rs and preparing adults to manipulate the external environment. During the last two decades, however, the public's fascination with Eastern studies has combined with a long-established undercurrent of interest among psychologists, awakening the medical profession to the trained mind's ability to promote health.

Among many psychological techniques applied to physical illness, the most widely used and successful has been the one called imaging or visualization. I will explain how it works and then present some examples, concentrating on health problems, that require nothing more than a quiet room and a friend or tape recorder. I will discuss relaxation, hypnosis, meditation, and visualization separately, but they are really all part of one process, as you'll understand when practicing them.

RELAXATION

By relaxation I don't mean falling asleep in front of the TV set or unwinding with friends. The kind I'm talking about is a quieting of mental activity and withdrawal of body and mind from external stimulation, a way of "erasing the blackboard" of all mundane concerns in preparation for contacting deeper layers of the mind. The goal is to reach a light trance state, sometimes called the alpha state because in it brain waves consist mainly of alpha waves, those whose frequency is between 8 and 12 cycles per second and which appear during deep relaxation. Inducing this state is the first step in hypnosis, biofeedback, yogic meditation, and most related forms of mind exploration.

There are many methods of relaxation, nearly all of them quite similar. They are thoroughly discussed, along with their physiological effects, in Dr. Herbert Benson's bestseller *The Relaxation Response,* one of the first books to approach the subject from a medical point of view.

One method differs somewhat from most of the others. Dr. Ainslie Meares of Melbourne, Australia, believes that all verbal instructions, even in the beginning, tend to stimulate too much logical thought. He has reported several remarkable regressions of cancer using a nonverbal quieting method based on gentle touching and reassuring sounds by the therapist. He also believes that best results depend on a slight degree of discomfort to be overcome by the patient, such as that produced by sitting on a low stool or straight-backed chair. Healing touch can certainly be significant when the patient has someone to administer it regularly, but other ways of inducing the relaxation response also achieve excellent results.

See the Appendix for a guided relaxation.

Don't be discouraged if you find relaxation procedures hard at first. Relaxation and meditation are perhaps especially difficult for Americans. Our constant mental diet of advertising, noise, violence, and media stimulation makes it very difficult to endure even a few minutes of inactivity and quiet. We have created a wall around ourselves to block out this deluge. In the process we also stop feeling and the quiet can be threatening. It gives us time to think and feel again.

MEDITATION

Someone once said, "Prayer is talking; meditation is listening." Actually it's a method by which we can temporarily *stop* listening to the pressures and distractions of everyday life and thereby are able to acknowledge other things—our deeper thoughts and feelings, the products of our unconscious mind, the peace of pure consciousness, and spiritual awareness.

To call it listening makes it sound entirely passive, but meditation is also an active process, although not in the usual sense. It is a way of focusing the mind in a state of relaxed awareness that, although less responsive to distractions, is more focused than usual toward things we want to pay attention to—images of healing, for example.

There are many ways of doing this. Some teachers recommend focusing your attention on a symbolic sound or word (a mantra), or on a single image, such as a candle flame or a mandala. Others focus on the relaxed ebb and flow of the breath, or gently restrain the mind from following the thoughts that flicker across its surface. The end of all the methods is ultimately the same: a deeply restful emptiness, or trance, that strengthens the mind by freeing it from its accustomed turmoil.

With guidance and practice, meditation can lead to breathtaking experiences of cosmic at-oneness and enlightenment, but the changes in the beginning are typically gentle and subtle. As you begin meditating, you'll find that it improves your concentration. Gradually you become centered within yourself, so that you no longer react so strongly to outside stresses. When someone cuts you off on the highway, you can avoid or shorten that hair-trigger surge of frustrated anger and its corresponding rise in blood pressure. The calmness also leaves you better prepared to avoid danger from other people's foolish actions.

I know of no other single activity that by itself can produce such a great improvement in the quality of life. I once received a letter from a group of women who began meditating to increase their breast size. Indeed, they were able to accomplish that, but the meditation experience itself so improved their lives that breast size became secondary and they became more interested in the complete revitalization that was taking place.

The physical benefits of meditation have recently been well documented by Western medical researchers, notably Dr. Herbert Benson. It tends to lower or normalize blood pressure, pulse rate, and the levels of stress hormones in the blood. It produces changes in brain-wave patterns, showing less excitability. These physical changes reflect changes in attitude, which show up on psychological tests as a reduction in the overcompetitive Type A behavior that increases the risk of heart attack. Meditation also raises the pain threshold and reduces one's biological age. Its benefits are multiplied when combined with regular exercise. In short, it reduces wear and tear on both body and mind, helping people live better and longer.

Western science has only just begun to study the effects of meditation and visualization on disease, although the interrelationships among the brain, endocrine glands, and immune system, as described in Chapter 3, are probably the way these effects occur. Perhaps the most direct research was a 1976 pilot study by Gurucharan Singh Khalsa, founder of Boston's Kundalini Research Institute. The study, conducted at the Veterans Administration hospital in La Jolla, California, showed that regular yoga and meditation increased blood levels of three important immune-system hormones by 100 percent. Unfortunately, this work could only be done with a few test subjects, and funds have not yet been granted to follow it up.

In 1980, however, psychologist Alberto Villoldo of San Francisco State College showed that regular meditation and self-healing visualization improved white-blood-cell response and improved the efficiency of hormone response to a standard test of physical stress—immersing one arm in ice water. The subjects trained in meditation withstood the pain of the test far better than those who did not meditate, and two-thirds of them were able to stop bleeding immediately after a blood test merely by focusing their minds on the vein after the needle was removed. This is easy to do, and I suggest that each of you try it the next time you have a blood sample drawn. Dr. Joan Borysenko, working at Boston's Beth Israel Hospital, has also shown that relaxation and meditation reduce the need for insulin among diabetics.

Type A individuals almost always are very competitive, have a great need to be in control, are inhibited by peer standards of behavior and emotional expression, and tend to get sick when the road to power is blocked or external rewards for their achievements are denied. Most of their goals involve gratifying their egos with externals, but they often short-change the more basic needs of their own bodies—perhaps because they tend to undervalue the egoless love and inner peace on which a feeling of self-worth ultimately depends. Type B individuals have a greater need for cooperation than power, are less inhibited, and more resistant to illness. This stage of development is reached by people whose primary motive is to give rather than to get, such as those parents who are able to turn from a primary concern with the self to a greater concern for their children. Paradoxically, this altruism—which is based on unconditional love rather than anticipated praise or other reward—reinforces a genuine self-esteem that enables people to care for themselves effectively. Both giver and receiver are rewarded by the act of love itself.

All the research to date indicates that the power drive, with its constant anxieties, continually activates the sympathetic (excitatory) part of the body's nervous system, with a consequent deactivation of the parasympathetic (calming) nerves. This in turn keeps the fight-or-flight stress response of adrenaline continually switched on, diminishing the body's ability to respond to another stress, such as illness. Harvard psychology professor David C. McClelland recently found that individuals motivated by power had lower levels of immunoglobulin A in their saliva than those motivated by concern for others. As McClelland has written, "This suggests that one way to avoid the stress and illness associated with a strong power drive is to grow up, to turn the power drive into helping others. Maturity, love, and detachment reduce sympathetic activation and its potentially bad effects on one's health."

There is nothing like meditation to give the calm and perspective needed for this growing up.

VISUALIZATION AND HYPNOSIS

Anthropologist Claude Lévi-Strauss has noted that much of folk medicine throughout the world is based on "psychological manipulation of the sick organ" by means of an extremely vivid image brought into the mind while the patient is in a deep trance. Carl and Stephanie Simonton adopted similar techniques learned from Mind Dynamics after hearing that users of biofeedback often were able to communicate more effectively with their bodies by means of an image than by directly trying to influence a certain organ or function. One woman, for example, learned to control a dangerous irregularity in her heartbeat by picturing a little girl swinging rhythmically to and fro on a playground swing.

In *Beyond Biofeedback,* Elmer and Alyce Green of the Menninger Clinic describe the experience of a close friend who was called in to help a man deal with the pain of a large pelvic cancer. The patient was hypnotized and asked to find the room in his brain that had the valves controlling the blood supply to his body and to turn off the valve that controlled the blood flow to his tumor. He did, and during two months of sessions the tumor shrank to one-fourth its former size. His pain went away, and he was discharged from the hospital instead of dying. Subsequently, when the man died because of a complication of later surgery, doctors found that his diffuse metastatic disease had disappeared, and his tumor, which had been the size of a grapefruit, was down to the size of a golf ball.

In a study reported in 1984, Dr. Nicholas Hall of the George Washington Medical Center in Washington, D.C., found that imaging increased the number of circulating white blood cells and also the levels of thymosin-alpha-1, a hormone especially important to the auxiliary white cells called T helper cells. Thymosin-alpha-1 also helps produce feelings of well-being, showing that the immune system can directly affect one's state of mind, as well as vice versa.

The Simontons were fortunate when they first helped a cancer patient use their visualization methods in 1971. Their initial subject was exceptionally imaginative and disciplined, and the results were better than anyone expected. The patient, a man with advanced throat cancer, had radiation for two months even though the specialists thought its chances of helping him were slim. But the patient visualized the treatment and his white blood cells in a positive way; he experienced no side effects and his cancer dramatically disappeared. He then went on to cure his arthritis and a twenty-year case of impotence using the imagery technique, all within four months. Such dramatic results enabled the Simontons to develop their method, knowing it could save lives, even though later patients did not always do as well. Often the first to receive a new treatment do very well because of the enhanced placebo effect. It is inherent in the intense interest, desires, and hope of the investigators.

Visualization takes advantage of what might almost be called a "weakness" of the body: it cannot distinguish between a vivid mental experience and an actual physical experience. Psychologist Charles Garfield studied cancer survivors at the University of California Medical Center in San Francisco and concluded that most of them had the ability to enter states of mind that enabled their bodies to perform, like those of athletes, at levels beyond the ordinary. Garfield found remarkable similarities between what the cancer survivors often did and the methods used by the Soviet and Eastern European competitors who have enjoyed such success in the Olympics during recent decades. These techniques, mainly developed in Bulgaria, have recently been described in detail by Sheila Ostrander and Lynn Schroeder in their book *Superlearning*.

Eastern European trainers often have their students and athletes lie down and listen to calming music, especially the largo movements of baroque instrumental music, with their strong, regular bass-line rhythms of about sixty beats per minute. After a few minutes, the listener's heartbeat becomes synchronized with the beat of the music, producing deep relaxation. Then the athlete visualizes, in full color and complete detail, a winning performance. This is repeated until the physical act becomes merely a duplication of a mental act that has already been successfully visualized. Soviet research indicates that athletes who spend as much as three-fourths of their time on mental training do better than those who place more emphasis on physical preparation.

Despite the Russian preference for baroque largos, many kinds of music work quite well, such as many types of classical music, gentle ballads, and spiritual music from any era or culture. Recordings of natural environments, such as the sea or bird songs in a forest, or even white noise like that of a waterfall, are also effective. The main concerns are that the sounds be quieting rather than stimulating and that they please the person who's hearing them. Besides using music in meditation, we begin each ECaP session with some calming music. This makes it easier to enter the state of "loving confrontation" we are trying to achieve. The music helps people relax and help each other face unpleasant truths, while remaining secure in the knowledge that we really care about each other.

Even though it may be helpful, however, you don't *need* music for visualization. As your concentration improves, you can do imaging meditation anywhere, even on a subway. Often the environmental noises can be woven into the imagery or hypnotic suggestion and help deepen the trance. The only requirement for effective visualization is development of your imagination. Seek specific help from a trained therapist if you have difficulty. We are not all visual and techniques for successful imagery or hypnosis vary. This is discussed further in the appendix.

The power of a vivid imagination struck me most clearly in the case of Garrett, a young child who had a brain tumor. It was inoperable, and following radiation treatments he still had his brain tumor. His doctors said there were no further tests or treatments that could help. His parents took him to the Biofeedback and Psychophysiology Center at the Menninger Clinic, where one of the staff taught him some self-regulation techniques—"how to control his body with his mind." The staff member had an imagery tape but he thought it was too boring for kids and wanted to make a tape that kids would like. Garrett decided he liked the idea of rocket ships, as in a video game, flying around in his head, shooting at the tumor. He imagined the cancer as "a big, round, dumb-looking thing" and blasted it regularly.

One night months later he told his father, "I can't find my tumor anymore." Though his father sat with him to help him concentrate, all he could see in his imagery was normal brain where his tumor used to be. Garrett wanted another CAT scan, but since the tumor was considered incurable, there seemed no reason to put him through the experience or expense. However after he fell down the stairs, a CAT scan was ordered to check for a skull fracture, and the tumor was shown to be entirely gone.

If we could just tell everybody, "Get out those rocket ships," the problem would be easy. Unfortunately, this technique doesn't always work. We just don't know enough about the process and how to individualize it and create change at an unconscious level of the mind.

From years of experience in using the visualization technique we do know that the image must be chosen by the individual. It must be an image that that person can see in the mind's eye as clearly as something seen by the physical eyes. It must be an image with which the patient feels completely comfortable. I believe one of the shortcomings of the Simontons' book is the absence of the spiritual aspects of healing. Since their initial patients were an aggressive group, they assumed that everyone would be comfortable attacking and killing cancer. A majority of people are profoundly disturbed by any picture of themselves killing anything, even an invading disease organism. The prevailing medical imagery of warfare is terribly upsetting to such people, even if they aren't conscious of it. Medical jargon words like *assault, insult, blast, poison,* and *kill* cause conscious and unconscious rejection by the patient. One ECaP patient, for example, a young man named Ian, listened to his oncologist tell him his treatment would kill his leukemia. Ian got up and left. On the way out, he said, "I'm a Quaker, a conscientious objector, and I don't kill *anything.*"

Ian entered individual and group psychotherapy, worked on developing a clear conscience, took twenty grams of vitamin C every day, meditated, and in general chose what was right for him. He visualized the appropriate immune-system cells gently carrying the cancerous cells away and instead of killing them flushing them out of the body. His disease slowly but steadily improved for four years. Then one winter he fell on the ice, hit his head, and suffered a concussion. He was told to lie down for a month. He used that month almost entirely for meditation and visualization. When he went for his regular checkup, his doctor told him, "This is the best blood count you've ever had." His wife said, "If we could just hit him in the head once a month, he'd probably get well."

As far as cancer is concerned, Ian's attitude is actually more realistic than the war model, because malignant cells are the body's own cells gone astray. In a sense, then, a direct attack is an attack on oneself. Moreover, most people feel comfortable about killing only out of love, in defense of loved ones, friends, family, or children. Psychological studies show that only about 15 percent of soldiers feel comfortable killing the enemy—unless they develop love for their comrades and think in terms of defending their loved ones.

But cancer patients often have had lifelong difficulty in loving themselves enough to feel the same way about self-defense. Thus some patients do well seeing their white blood cells as sharks or polar bears, but many do not. Some of the most successful kinds of visualization in ECaP have been images of tumors as *food*, being eaten by white cells disguised as Pac-Men or some such benevolent consumer. Just as healers in primitive tribes tell people to utilize power animals, I suggest that patients use similar animated symbols. One child saw his cancer as cat food and immune cells as white pussycats. Another patient visualized birds and birdseed. One lady who had oat-cell cancer pictured mares and does eating her oats. Seeing the cancer as being eaten can mean "This tumor will nourish me and help me get well." This kind of picture is truer to the real nature of the white blood cells and also offers a framework for using the disease as psychological food for one's own growth. Another comfortable image is seeing the disease as a delinquent, or misbehaving child or body part. Through treatment and discipline the abnormal part or disease is returned to normal, mature function.

For guided visualization techniques, see the Appendix.

7

You cannot teach a man anything. You can only
help him to find it within himself.

—GALILEO

Images in Disease and Healing

I began working with imagery and cancer using the approach developed by the Simontons and specifically outlined by their co-workers Jeanne Achterberg and Frank Lawlis in *Imagery of Cancer* (now expanded and titled *Imagery of Disease*). Using these techniques, I, too, found consistent differences between the images of patients who would do well compared with those who would do poorly. The differences showed up in such pictorial elements as the bulk of the cancer, the aggressiveness of white blood cells, and the ways in which treatment was symbolized.

I had used this method for a year in a rather mechanical way to try to direct patients toward healing. Then, in the fall of 1979, I participated in a Life-Death Transition workshop run by Elisabeth Kübler-Ross. The drawings I made as part of that workshop (see example in insert following page 116) helped me reach a deeper understanding of the powerful relationship between one's unconscious and one's emotional life.

These techniques for using drawings to explore the unconscious have been developed over many decades by Carl Jung's student Susan Bach, and by Gregg Furth and others. I learned them from Dr. Kübler-Ross, and as I applied them in my practice, I saw that there were patterns of color symbolism and that time sequences of past, present, and future were often revealed. However, I saw that the symbol associations were often as complex and revealing as dreams.

Back in 1933, Jung interpreted the following dream submitted to him by a doctor who provided no other information about the patient:

Someone beside me kept asking me something about oiling some machinery. Milk was suggested as the best lubricant. Apparently I thought that oozy slime was preferable. Then, a pond was drained and amid the slime there were two extinct animals. One was a minute mastodon. I forgot what the other one was.

Jung correctly diagnosed a damming-up of cerebrospinal fluid probably due to a tumor. His interpretation was based on the facts that the Latin word for phlegm, one kind of bodily "slime," is *pituita*, and that "mastodon" derives from two Greek words meaning "breast" and "teeth." He deduced that the mastodon image referred to the mammillary bodies, breast-shaped structures lying at the bottom of the third ventricle, a "pond" of cerebrospinal fluid at the base of the brain.

The details of Jung's interpretation are brilliantly recaptured by UCLA research psychologist Russell Lockhart in his article "Cancer in Myth and Dream." When asked how he had arrived at the correct conclusion, Jung himself only replied:

. . . why I must take that dream as an organic symptom would start such an argument that you would accuse me of the most terrible obscurantism. . . . When I speak of archetypal patterns those of you who are aware of these things understand, but if you are not you think, "This fellow is absolutely crazy because he talks of mastodons and their difference from snakes and horses." I should have to give you a course of about four semesters about symbology first so that you could appreciate what I said.

As Lockhart concluded, "Bodily organs and processes have the capacity to stimulate the production of psychic images, meaningfully related to the type of physical disturbance and its location." This probably comes about by means of electrical and/or chemical messages from the diseased part of the body to the brain, which are interpreted by the mind as images. Just as a salamander cannot grow a new limb if the nerves to it have been cut, so we cannot receive these messages if the nervous system is damaged or if our minds are closed to conscious communication with psyche and soma.

As you can see, a great deal of knowledge about language and mythology is often necessary to interpret dreams correctly. Like Jung, I believe that the mind has available to it the experience of all previous life. This is why people sometimes dream in languages consciously unknown to them, or in a universal language of symbols whose meanings they do not know when awake. Drawings are easier to interpret, because the symbolism is generally simpler, more closely related to everyday life, and can be directed to a specific theme.

I ask my patients to draw themselves, their treatment, their disease, and their white cells eliminating the disease. To elicit undirected material from the unconscious, I ask each patient for at least one additional drawing of a scene of his or her own choosing. Depending on what areas of conflict exist, I may also ask them to draw themselves at work, at home with their family, in the operating room, and so on.

One of the conflicts I most often see concerns the patient's attitude toward treatment. On a conscious or intellectual level the patient is often saying, "This treatment is good for me," yet unconsciously feeling, "This is poison." In such a case, there is only one way out: if the patient reacts as though poisoned, treatment must be stopped. However, once a drawing reveals a patient's resistance to treatment, that attitude can be changed. It can be made conscious and dealt with. It requires the visualization of successful therapy, a reprogramming at an unconscious level.

I discuss the drawings with each patient, sometimes for hours, before the first ECaP session or as part of the consultation before surgery. The drawings are a wonderful way to get people to open up and talk about things they would otherwise conceal. After all, *they* have made the picture, and the conflicts and attitudes it represents are now there on paper for both of us to see. Furthermore, it doesn't matter how many of my lectures a patient has attended, or how much he or she knows about the picture-drawing technique. The unconscious always knows more symbols and finds new ways of revealing something that consciousness has concealed.

Susan Bach has worked with this approach for over thirty

years, much of that time in children's hospitals where the use
of drawings was encouraged. She has found specific illnesses
reflected in a typical, recurrent way.

She writes:

We may comprehend that the human being can and does
convey, through these wordless communications and in his own
idiom, both his somatic and his psychological condition.
Somatically, such pictures may point to events in the past
relevant to anamnesis [recall], early diagnosis, and prognosis.
Psychologically, we may see what goes on and has been going on
deep in the mind—for instance, past traumas—and how the
drawing can help him to express his hopes, fear, and forebodings.
Moreover, these pictures can build a bridge between doctor and
patient, the family, and the surrounding world. Indeed, their
meaning and what it implies could guide the healing profession to
assist especially the critically ill patient in living as near to his
essential being as possible, whether in recovery or before his life's
circle closes.

Finally, we may ask how it could be that spontaneous
pictures reflect, as dreams do, the total situation of the human
person. I have come to see, in decades of clinical work, that
through the imagery of spontaneous pictures and of dreams
something shines through, which I have called "inner
knowingness." Thus a new dimension may be opening before us.

In her own way, psychologist Joan Kellogg has shown that
patient drawings of mandalas, an ancient Indian type of circular symbolic image representing wholeness or one's whole life,
can reveal much about the unconscious life of the mind. The
person fills in a circular outline with colored geometric designs
or pictures, which are then interpreted in a dialogue with the
healer or therapist.

For examples of drawings by patients, see the insert following page 116. They have been chosen to illustrate some of
the things this technique can reveal. I have made no attempt
to give a complete interpretation of each picture. Nor have I
tried to teach the art of interpretation itself, which would
require an entire book.

8

Becoming Exceptional

Psychologist Al Siebert became interested in the personalities of survivors when he joined the paratroopers just after college in 1953. His training cadre consisted of the few survivors of a unit that had been virtually wiped out in Korea. He found these veterans to be tough but more patient than he'd expected. In response to mistakes they usually made a joke instead of getting angry. More important, Siebert wrote, "I observed that they had a relaxed awareness. Each one seemed to have a sort of personal radar that was always on scan." He realized that it wasn't primarily luck that had brought these men through their ordeal.

Throughout his career Siebert has continued to study survivors. He has found that one of their most prominent characteristics is a complexity of character, a union of many opposites that he has termed biphasic traits. They are both serious *and* playful, tough *and* gentle, logical *and* intuitive, hard-working *and* lazy, shy *and* aggressive, introspective *and* outgoing, and so forth. They are paradoxical people who don't fit neatly into the usual psychological categories. This makes them more flexible than most people, with a wider array of resources to draw upon.

Siebert wondered how the survivor personality keeps from being immobilized by its contradictions. Building on concepts of Ruth Benedict and Abraham Maslow, and interviewing hundreds of people who had lived through all kinds of hardships, Siebert found that survivors have a hierarchy of needs and that, unlike most people, they pursue *all* of them. Beginning with the most basic, these needs are: survival, safety, acceptance by others, self-esteem, and self-actualization. One of the main needs that distinguished survivors from others, however, went beyond self-actualization: a need for synergy. Siebert defines the need for synergy as the need to have things work well for oneself *and* others.

Survivors, then, act not only from self-interest but also from the interest of others, even in the most stressful situations. They clean up messes and make things safer or more efficient. In short, they give of themselves, leaving the world better than they found it. Their relaxed awareness and the confidence that it brings allow them to save their energies for the really important things. When things are going well, they let well enough alone, leaving themselves free for curiosity about new developments or potential problems. They may seem uninvolved at times, but they are "foul-weather friends." They show up when there's trouble.

SURVIVORS OF ILLNESS

Siebert's survival characteristics are remarkably similar to those of patients who do well in the Simonton program and in ECaP. The Simontons have summarized the psychological profile of their exceptional patients as follows: They are generally successful at careers they like, and they remain employed during illness or return to work soon. They are receptive and creative, but sometimes hostile, having strong egos and a sense of their own adequacy. They have a high degree of self-esteem and self-love. They are rarely docile. They retain control of their lives. They are intelligent, with a strong sense of reality. They are self-reliant: they don't *need* to be included among others although they *value* interactions with others. Although concerned with their own welfare, they are also tolerant and concerned with others. They tend to be nonconformists with a permissive morality—they are unprejudiced, and they appreciate diversity among other people.

As patients, those who have or are developing survival

traits are self-reliant and seek solutions rather than lapsing into depression. They interpret problems as redirections, not failures. They are the ones who read or meditate in the waiting room instead of staring forlornly into space. As an ECaP member once put it, "Pessimism is a luxury I can't afford." One cancer patient vomited so frequently during her course of radiation treatments that she couldn't absorb enough food to keep herself nourished. So she set the alarm for 4 A.M. every day, had breakfast then, and had lunch at 8 A.M. That way she had two meals digested before her afternoon treatment, and her vitality was restored.

Our goal in ECaP is to help people live by developing the resilience, adaptability, and confidence of the survivor personality. One of my patients told me she'd asked her doctor whether anybody ever got over what she had. I confronted her with the question "If you were in a concentration camp, would you ask a guard, 'Does anybody ever get out of here?' " It turned out that she'd been in a concentration camp, so she knew exactly what I was talking about.

Just as negativity feeds on itself, so does the positive outlook of a survivor, and the body reflects the mind. When I went on the Phil Donahue Show with three ECaP members in April of 1979, a makeup man came into our crowded dressing room, looked around, and asked, "Okay, who are the cancer patients?" I guess he expected three green women. He simply couldn't tell, and that was one of the best psychotherapy sessions these patients ever had, an enormous boost to their sense of well-being.

One of these three ECaP women met a former boyfriend in Chicago, stayed, and married him. She chose not to have radiation therapy for her breast cancer. She is alive and well today, and I feel that her remarriage and the redirection of her life helped save her. One of the others, who has had cancer twice, is also free of the disease today.

The third patient, named Melanie, later died—but not of cancer, rather from a treatment complication, an infection after a bone-marrow transplant. Her story began during a divorce when her husband asked her how she was doing. She said, "I'm having a very difficult time," and he said, "Oh, you look terrific." She thought, "I'll never share anything with him again." She held all her feelings inside and developed leukemia. She made a very significant change in her lifestyle thereafter. Many times, when her physicians thought she would not survive, she did. This happened so often that later on, when it *really* looked as though she wouldn't survive, her physicians reinforced her beliefs by telling her they expected her to recover, and she did once more. Melanie got to the point where she literally ran out of chemotherapy options, because she had so many remissions. Finally, she underwent a bone-marrow transplant, which is not usual in someone as old as she. (She was in her thirties.) I sent a letter to the hospital, explaining what an exceptional patient she was. They accepted her and learned from her that age alone is not the significant issue, but rather your will to live and survival characteristics.

One of the most heartening aspects of ECaP's work is the way our members can often help each other. Recently one of my patients told me she'd had a call from her brother, who was facing serious back surgery. She gave him a lesson in how to behave as an exceptional patient, and a few days later he called her again to say he was being discharged on the sixth day, even though his doctor had told him he'd be in for twelve to twenty-four.

Siebert, too, has found that the survivor personality can be learned—although it can't be "taught" the way algebra or chemistry can. He conceives of it as a broad process of psychological and neurological maturation, a growing up that paradoxically involves remaining a child, too. It means being child-like but not childish. Siebert lists the following indicators of self-motivated growth:

- Aimless playfulness for its own sake, like that of a happy child.
- The ability to become so deeply absorbed in an activity that you lose track of time, external events, and all your worries, often whistling, humming, or talking to yourself absent-mindedly.
- A child's innocent curiosity.
- An observant, nonjudgmental style.

- Willingness to look foolish, make mistakes, and laugh at yourself.
- Open-minded acceptance of criticism about yourself.
- An active imagination, daydreams, mental play, and conversations with yourself.

Seibert has also identified the following signs that show a person is reaching the synergistic level of functioning:

- Empathy for other people, including opponents.
- The ability to see patterns and relationships in organizations or equipment.
- Recognition of subliminal perception or intuition as a valid source of information.
- Good timing, especially when speaking or taking an original action.
- The ability to see early clues about future developments and take appropriate action.
- Cooperative nonconformity: refusing to be controlled by improper laws or social standards, yet choosing to abide by them most of the time for the sake of others—unless attempting to change them. In other words, an avoidance of empty gestures.
- Being comfortable in complex, confusing situations that others find bewildering and frightening.
- Keeping a positive outlook and confidence in adversity.
- The ability to absorb new, unexpected, or unpleasant experiences and be changed by them.
- A talent for serendipity: the ability to convert what others consider accidents or misfortunes into something useful.
- The feeling of getting smarter and enjoying life more as you get older.*

If interpreted as a set of goals, this list may seem formidable, but as I discuss the major ones in the rest of this chapter, I hope to show that they develop automatically from personal

---

*For more information about the survivor personality and the synergy need, write to Al Siebert, P.O. Box 535, Portland, Oregon 97207.

growth toward expressing love, both self-love *and* love for others. And, although personality change is hard, you *can* make each of these traits your own. This doesn't happen simply by wishing, however. There are two major ways to make the changes easier: By working within a supportive therapy group or by sharing honestly with your most trusted loved ones, you can confront your habits and behavior. A friend has called this process "carefrontation," to combine the love and confrontation in one word. The second way of facilitating these changes is by regular meditation in which you visualize yourself as you want to become. This helps you work at the unconscious level of the mind, where all meaningful change occurs, rather than just on the conscious level of awareness.

SELF-RESPECT AND CREATIVITY

"What matters is what you think about yourself. You must find the part in life that fits you and then give up acting; your profession is being." So wrote Quentin Crisp, the English author and lecturer who calls himself a "retired waif" on his tax returns and chronicled his long journey to self-acceptance in *The Naked Civil Servant.* When they were boys, his brothers wanted to be football players and ships' captains. He wanted to be a chronic invalid. Until Crisp "gave up acting," he actually was a chronic invalid. After he stopped worrying what other people might think about his eccentric dress, gay lifestyle, brightly dyed hair, and gently subversive opinions, he became robustly healthy, taking long and hectic speaking tours in his stride well into his seventies.

Emotional honesty and self-acceptance lead to better physical health, as science is beginning to document. In 1979, for example, Drs. Walter Smith and Stephen Bloomfield found that people who can cry freely catch fewer colds than people who always hold back their tears. These are realities that women tend to understand better than men, for women are more used to accepting and working with their emotions, while men's lives tend to revolve around their work. This is no doubt why ECaP groups so far have been composed mainly of women. And women have better survival rates for the same cancer than men.

Psychologists estimate that less than 20 percent of the population has an "inner locus of control," the kind of self-possession in which persons are guided by their own standards rather than beliefs about what others may think. This integrity is a large part of the survivor personality, and the percentage is the same as the percentage of exceptional patients I've found among patients in general. As Elida Evans observed in her groundbreaking 1926 study of the cancer personality, "Development of individuality is a safeguard to life and health. It lifts a person out of the collective authority." I find in rural or rugged areas the percentage of exceptional patients is higher. They are independent, self-reliant people to begin with.

Becoming your own person releases your creativity. Freed from the bonds of convention and the fear of what others may think, the mind responds with new solutions, new goals, and an awareness that beauty and peace come from within. You become able to take risks, to experiment with your own life.

In his memoirs *Most of All, They Taught Me Happiness,* Robert Müller recounts an extreme example of the survivor's ability to think creatively under pressure. In 1943 Müller was a member of the French Resistance. Using the name Parizot, he had infiltrated an agency of the Vichy government, where he gathered information on German troop movements. Tipped off that the Nazis had just driven up to arrest him, he fled to the attic of his office building. Word came that half a dozen Gestapo men, knowing he was there, were methodically searching the premises.

Müller had been following Dr. Émile Coué's program of autosuggestion and positive thinking. He had been introduced to this method by a friend who had been hospitalized with tuberculosis and told that he would not survive the disease. He had asked Müller to bring him books by Coué, and Müller had read them, too. His friend had recovered from the tuberculosis, inspiring Müller's belief in Coué's system.

By repeating to himself that the situation could be seen as a thrilling adventure, Müller calmed himself enough to realize the one thing the Nazis would not expect him to do—walk downstairs to meet them.

By taking off his glasses, slicking down his hair with water, grabbing a file folder from a vacant desk, and lighting a cigarette, Parizot managed to change his appearance somewhat and assume an air of calm. Walking downstairs, he came upon his secretary as she was being interrogated. He asked her what all the excitement was about. Without batting an eye, she said the "gentlemen" were looking for Mr. Parizot. "Parizot?" he exclaimed. "But I just saw him a few minutes ago on the fourth floor!" The Nazis rushed upstairs, and Müller was led to safety by his friends.

Few of us are put to such a direct test, but we all have the opportunity to live inventively. People who develop their full individuality often change jobs, moving from a career that bores them but gives them security into one that brings meaning to their lives and provides them with a way of giving something to the world rather than just getting something from it. The late Senator Frank Church of Idaho, for example, was in Harvard Law School in 1947 when he was diagnosed as having incurable cancer and given six months to live. Then he found another doctor who prescribed the then-new radiation treatment that started his cure.

In an interview three decades later, Church described his decision to enter politics to try to do some good for other people: "I had previously tended to be more cautious—but having so close a brush with death at 23, I felt afterwards that life itself is such a chancy proposition that the only way to live it is by taking great chances." As a result, he was not afraid to be the first senator to publicly oppose the Vietnam War, to investigate CIA and FBI crimes, and to sponsor politically dangerous civil-rights and environmental legislation. His own defeat and the repudiation of his ideals in the conservative landslide of 1980 may have contributed to his death from cancer in 1984, thirty-seven years after the original prognosis.

There's no question that job satisfaction is important to health. As Hans Selye, the world's greatest authority on stress, has pointed out, "If you do what you like, you never really work. Your work is your play." Somebody once came upon

George Halas, owner of the Chicago Bears football team, sitting in his office on a weekend. He asked Halas, then in his eighties, "George, at your age, what are you doing here working?" Halas replied, "It's only work if there's someplace else you'd rather be."

The person suffering in an unsatisfying career often argues that there aren't enough interesting, creative jobs to go around. This may be true, but so few people exercise their creativity that the opportunities exist for those who seek them. Nothing can be gained without effort, and, as William James noted, most people live too far within self-imposed limits.

There is a seeming contradiction here that traps many people. Most of us have been taught that self-love and love for others are incompatible, that we can't satisfy our own needs and still give of ourselves. If we become survivors, we realize that our deepest need *is* to love and be at peace and, our motivation becomes spiritual or selfless, not selfish. Living with the knowledge that we're going to die someday means that we may choose to give something to the world. In the process, we develop an inner sense of worth that helps us achieve goals that improve the quality of life. We find ourselves striving for the survivor's paradoxical goal—to have things work out well for ourselves *and* others.

People who suffer in unsatisfying jobs are assuming the victim role. Nothing is going to help them if they don't help themselves. Too much is made of work defined as a job, anyway. People often come into my office and say, "I'd like to be a therapist. Where can I do this work?" I say, "Where do you work now?" When they tell me, I say, "Okay, now look around you, and you'll find that everyone in that office has pain. Help them, and you'll immediately become a therapist." A patient of mine named Ted, who eight years ago developed two brain tumors, one malignant and one benign, put it this way: "I used to be a miserable son of a bitch. I used to install carpets, and I would tell people, 'All I want is money.' Now what I do [hospital volunteer work] is free, and I love it."

Stephanie Matthews has said, "The biggest obstacle we have to get over is the idea that work is the only meaningful purpose in life—or for some women it's supposed to be their children." This is another area where meditation and visualization can be of enormous help. A person can temporarily disconnect from the pressures and unhappiness of the present job, and image a more congenial future. Imaging channels mental energy toward making the desired result happen, and as you begin to act upon your new awareness, you create new opportunities—both consciously and unconsciously.

We prepare our future by what we think and do each day. I recommend that patients keep a diary of their thoughts. As they read it later, they will see how they prepared their future by their thoughts, which then motivated their activities. Jung said, "The future is unconsciously prepared long in advance, and therefore can be guessed by clairvoyants."

In ECaP we help people, living with the uncertainty of illness, define their reasons for living. Many patients resist this effort, feeling there's no point in creating goals they may not live to carry out. And it certainly does take great courage, for when life is joyous, the loss seems greater. We are trying to get people to take on life as an exciting challenge and see it as a gift or an opportunity to do something.

I was recently called by Howard, a gentleman who'd been told by his doctor he'd be dead in three months. He went home, sat down in the living room and told his wife to cancel his dental appointments. His wife said, "I'm not going to have you sitting around the living room for three months dying." He came to me all the way from Montana. I said, "Anybody who comes here from Montana is not going to die in three months. You're different. You're a fighter." Eighteen months later, Howard is still alive. Written up in his hometown paper and shown meditating in his hot tub. His doctor said, "Boy, you're lucky." He said, "It's not luck. It's hard work." But he said the thing that turned him around was my saying, "You're different." I try to help people realize that it's the process of moving toward a goal that is important. As we change and work toward sainthood, the body benefits. The process is the product.

When we're setting goals in ECaP, we try not to get stuck in a time frame. This sets us up for failure if we don't accomplish our aims on schedule. The object is to help patients set *realistic* targets. Achievement of them reinforces feelings of competence and self-worth, and the goals themselves immediately make the future a brighter prospect. As Nietzsche wrote, "He who has a 'why' to live can bear almost any 'how.'" The ultimate goal is simply to live for ourselves, in a selfless way.

We help patients work toward a balanced set of goals that reflect all of their needs. Many people, especially men, tend to think only in terms of work-related goals, while many women tend to set goals having to do with others—such as getting a child through college or finishing a charity drive—to the exclusion of their own needs.

We encourage people to consider work, physical development, emotional and spiritual needs, help to others, and pure play when they set their goals—in other words, to integrate all aspects of their lives. It's especially important to know what needs have been met by the illness and to set goals that meet those needs in place of the illness.

Once again, meditation and visualization are powerful tools to help you be aware of your true needs and then make them happen. Seeing what you want in your mind's eye helps convince your unconscious that it's possible, and that helps create an atmosphere of hope. You are now receiving a "live" message.

The process of restructuring your life, of becoming an authentic person, means ceasing to think of yourself as a thing —a collection of habits, a job, a role. This is being a slave of your self-image and, in a sense, already dead. Instead we try to help patients understand themselves as dynamic, ever-changing processes. This comes about by recognizing that we are all perfectly imperfect. We are all bound by the inevitability of death and the fact that certain choices may speed the destructive processes. Nor do we know exactly when we will die, and within that uncertainty we all have almost unlimited options.

From a scientific viewpoint George T. Lock Land, in his book *Grow or Die,* has shown how our human condition is much like what we've learned about all living cells:

The nature of a cell, just like what we call "human nature," is not something that *is,* but something forever in the process of *becoming.* It is not wholly determined, but plays a great part in determining itself. As the human recapitulates the same series of events that take place in the life of a cell, his behavior depends on the alternatives available for growth. If the conditions of nutrition and feedback permit new growth patterns, the result will be creative and responsible behavior. If not, the *lack of alternatives results in a regression to more basic growth patterns.*

From an artistic point of view, Robert Henri has described the same kind of growth in *The Art Spirit:*

When the artist is alive in any person, whatever his kind of work may be, he becomes an inventive, searching, daring, self-expressive creature. He becomes interesting to other people. He disturbs, upsets, enlightens, and opens ways for a better understanding. Where those who are not artists are trying to close the book, he opens it and shows there are still more pages possible.

INDEPENDENCE AND ASSERTIVENESS

People who always smile, never tell anyone their troubles, and neglect their own needs are the ones who are most likely to become ill. For them, the main problem often is learning to say no without guilt. Many only become able to live for themselves, to tell others what they really feel, after the shock of the diagnosis. One patient, who never expressed displeasure at *anything,* began to improve when she was able to tell her husband that she didn't like the family dog. For Thelma, whom I mentioned in Chapter 2, the first milestone of growth came when, for once in her life, she walked out of the house with the phone ringing, and when she finally called the police when her alcoholic husband threatened her.

The most important kind of assertiveness a patient can demonstrate is in the formation of a participatory relationship with the doctor. Most patients don't talk to their doctors or ask a lot of questions for fear of angering this person who is going to "make" them well. Of course, no one can make you well. You heal. Many people get well while using alternative therapies. This does not necessarily mean that the therapy itself is useful, but that people heal doing something they believe in, something that gives them hope. That's what we help people learn in ECaP, and it often means helping doctors learn the same lesson. One morning on rounds a patient asked me, "What's wrong?"

"Nothing," I said.

"Then why are you frowning?"

"I'm not frowning, just thinking."

"Well, do your thinking in the hallway and smile in here." Our patients are our best teachers.

When a nurse tells me that some patient is being uncooperative, refusing to get undressed and put on the standard hospital gown, or asking all sorts of questions before submitting to a test, I say, "Fine. He'll live longer." And Leonard Derogatis's work mentioned in Chapter 1, showing that long-term survivors had "poorer" attitudes as judged by physicians, supports what I've observed on the wards. The so-called "problem patient" is also the rapid healer, the long-term survivor, and the one with the active immune system. That's why I encourage people to behave as individuals when they enter a hospital, by following this list of suggestions, which my wife and I call "Good Patient, Bad Patient":

1. For your hospital stay, take clothes that are practical, comfortable, and individual. Plan to walk as much as possible.

2. Take room decorations of a personal and inspirational nature. Make sure your room has a view of the sky and the outside world. Do not accept a room that faces a brick wall.

3. Question authority—tests, etc. Speak up for yourself, your needs and comfort in all areas, both before and during tests.

4. Make your doctor aware of your unique needs and desires. Offer to share books, tapes, and conversation.

5. Take tape recorder and earphones, along with meditation tapes and some of your favorite music. Record conversations with your physician for later review and for family use.

6. Use your tape recorder in the operating room and recovery room to hear music, meditation, or messages during and after surgery. Have someone put a reminder into the doctor's orders to play the entire tape continuously.

7. If you are having an operation, instruct the surgeon and anesthesiologist to repeat positive messages to you. The simplest is that you will awaken comfortable, thirsty, and hungry.

8. Tell the surgeon to speak to you during surgery, honestly but hopefully, and also to repeat positive messages but absolutely avoid negative ones.

9. Speak to your own body, particularly the night before surgery, suggesting that the blood leave the area of surgery and that you'll heal rapidly.

10. Arrange visits and calls from those who will nurture and love you, as well as give you carefrontation when appropriate.

11. Get moving as soon as possible after surgery. Leave the hospital to attend group meetings, go for walks, or have meals out with friends.

Honest expression of your feelings can make a big difference in the quality of care you receive. Emma, one of our exceptional patients, was depressed by the gray of her oncologist's waiting room, so one day she stood up and said, "This place is morbid. You can't get well here, and I don't want anybody here to sign insurance forms until this place is redecorated."

The secretary came out and said, "You can't do that."

Emma simply replied, "It's done." And the office was repainted blue. Now Emma is "the woman who made us redecorate our office." She's treated like a human being, not a disease.

Emma had lung nodules and asked her physician, "How do you know that those nodules are due to cancer rather than heartworm?" (Heartworm is a parasitic disease of dogs that is prevalent in Connecticut.)

The doctor answered, "Ninety-nine times out of a hundred they're due to cancer."

She persisted: "How do you *know?*" When he said he couldn't be sure, she demanded, "Do some tests." Blood tests showed a strong possibility that the nodules *were* heartworm, which recent statistics showed was especially common in the town where she lived.

Now Emma's doctor began to sound like her. He called a chest surgeon and said, "I have a patient with lung nodules, and I don't know whether they're due to heartworm or cancer."

The surgeon replied, "Ninety-nine times out of a hundred they're due to cancer." But her doctor requested more tests to be sure. Emma's self-assertiveness had created a new, more effective doctor-patient relationship.

THE FOUR FAITHS

Phyllis, a patient who had an extensive pancreatic cancer that was no longer responding to treatment, went home to die. Several months later she returned to the office. One of my partners examined her. He opened the door of the examining room and called me: "Hey, Bernie, you're interested in this stuff."

I came in, and he said, "Her cancer's gone."

"Phyllis," I said, "Tell them what happened."

She said, "Oh, you know what happened."

"I know that I know," I said, "but I'd like the others to know."

Phyllis replied, "I decided to live to be a hundred and leave my troubles to God."

I could really end the book here, because this peace of mind can heal anything. I believe faith is the essence, a simple solution, yet too hard for most people to practice.

To verify this I went to God (surgeons have that prerogative) and asked why I couldn't hang a sign in my waiting room saying, "Leave your troubles to God, you don't need me." God said, "I'll show you why. I'll meet you at the hospital at 10 A.M. Saturday." (God likes to play doctor.) On Saturday he said, "Take me to your sickest patient." I told him about a woman with cancer whose husband had run off with another woman. He said, "Good case," and we went up to her room. I said, "Ma'am, God is going to come in and tell you how to get well." I always introduce him so patients are not overwhelmed. She responded, "Oh, wonderful." God entered the room and said, "All you have to do is love, accept, forgive, and choose to be happy," and she looked Him in the eye and said, "Have you met my husband yet?" Most of us want God to change the external aspects of our lives so we don't have to change internally. We want to be exempt from the responsibility for our own happiness. We often find it easier to resent and suffer in the role of victim than to love, forgive, accept, and find inner peace. As W. H. Auden has written,

> We would rather be ruined than changed;
> We would rather die in our dread
> Than climb the cross of the moment
> And let our illusions die.

Yet, when we choose to love, healing energy is released in our bodies. Energy itself is loving and intelligent and available to all of us.

Now I felt I had a dilemma: If God's love could cure people, I wondered, why should I remain a surgeon? So I returned to Him and said, "God, you know one of my patients got well leaving her troubles to you. Why should I remain a surgeon?" Why not just teach people to love?" And God in His beautiful, sweet, melodious voice said to me, "Bernie, render unto the surgeon what is the surgeon's, and render unto God what is God's." (I find that God does that a lot—speaks in parables and leaves you totally confused.) Since then I've come to understand that God and I both have a role in getting people well.

Let me illustrate what I mean with an old story I've adapted. A man with cancer is told by his primary physician he'll be dead in an hour. He runs to the window, looks up at the sky, and says, "God, save me." Out of the blue comes that wonderful melodious voice, saying, "Don't worry, my son. I will save you." The man climbs back into bed, feeling reassured.

His physician called me and I walk in, and say, "If I operate in an hour, I can save you." "No, thanks," says the man, "God will save me." Then an oncologist, a radiation therapist and a nutritional therapist all tell him, "We can save you." "I don't need you. God will save me," was his reply to all of them.

In an hour the man dies. When he gets to heaven, he walks up to God and says, "What happened? You said you'd save me, and here I am, dead."

"You dumbbell. I sent you a surgeon, an oncologist, a radiation therapist, and a nutritional therapist." There is a role for the mechanic when he is the patient's choice of therapy. I can be God's gift and tool also just as the bible states medication is.

In ECaP we've found that four faiths are crucial to recovery from serious illness: faith in oneself, one's doctor, one's treatment, and one's spiritual faith. We have discussed the first three, but the last, although seldom totally achievable by most of us, is in many ways a key to the others.

The "spiritual life" has many meanings. It need not be reflected in any commitment to an organized religion, and we all know that some of the most outwardly pious people are the least spiritual. These are the ones who give other people "spiritual ulcers," as a participant in one of my workshops phrased it. From the standpoint of a healer, I view spirituality as including the belief in some meaning or order in the universe. I view the force behind creation as a loving, intelligent energy. For some, this is labeled God, for others it can be seen simply as a source of healing. From this there comes the ability to find peace, to resolve the apparent contradictions between one's emotions and reality, between internal and external. Spirituality means acceptance of what is (not to be confused with resignation or approval of evil). Jesus told us to love our enemies, not like them and not have no enemies. In an abandoned, bombed-out house in Germany at the end of World War II, Allied soldiers found a testimony to this faith scratched into a basement wall by one of the victims of the Holocaust:

I believe in the sun—even when it does not shine;
I believe in love—even when it is not shown;
I believe in God—even when he does not speak.

Spirituality means the ability to find peace and happiness in an imperfect world, and to feel that one's own personality is imperfect but acceptable. From this peaceful state of mind come both creativity and the ability to love unselfishly, which go hand in hand. Acceptance, faith, forgiveness, peace, and love are the traits that define spirituality for me. These characteristics *always* appear in those who achieve unexpected healing of serious illness.

Most physicians won't "try God" until the patient is near death. Then they may prescribe a hope and a prayer. I believe it's far better to make a connection with the patient's spiritual beliefs earlier, when the job is easier. Anyone who believes that the world is basically a beautiful place—even if it came about because of Nature rather than God—has a reason to remain in it. A person who believes in a benevolent higher power has a potent reason for hope—and hope is physiologic.

Obviously, the "medical meaning" of religion varies from person to person. Those who profess a faith merely because their parents did or because it increases their social standing are unlikely to really believe it can heal them. Sometimes religion even becomes a negative factor. People think, "If God gave me this illness, who am I to get well?" Beliefs that lean heavily on guilt, original sin, and predestination are of little use for healing. By the same token, it's hard to find peace in life if you believe death is a meaningless end or earthly existence is futile. That's why I prefer to speak of spirituality rather than religion, to avoid doctrinal limitations. It's essential not to force a stereotyped picture of God on anyone. In ECaP we seek instead to use what is positive in each patient's beliefs.

I want to emphasize here the difference between wishing, which is passive, and hope, which is active. Hoping means seeing that the outcome you want is possible, and then working for it. Wishing means just sitting there, waiting for a miracle to happen out of the blue. Jung said, "Every problem, therefore, brings the possibility of a widening of consciousness, but also the necessity of saying goodbye to childlike unconsciousness and trust in nature," a process he likened to leaving the Garden of Eden. I encourage patients to have faith in God but not to expect Him to do all the work.

I think of God as the same potential healing force—an intelligent, loving energy or light—in each person's life. Even scientists are now telling us that energy has intelligence. Physicist Carl Pribram has said, "The universe must be friendly. It gave us physics, so we can understand what all those who preceded us already knew." I suggest that patients think of illness not as God's will but as our deviation from God's will. To me it is the absence of spirituality that leads to difficulties. I know that many patients, when they develop an illness or have a recurrence, are angry at God. It's important to be able to argue with God, as is traditional in Judaism. Continued helpless rage at the universe can't possibly lead to health. God isn't sitting up there with a clipboard, saying, "Let's see who I can make trouble for today." On the contrary, God is a resource. The energy of hope and faith is always available. We all must die someday, but the spiritual way is always open to everyone and can make our lives beautiful whenever we choose it. As German dramatist Christian Friedrich Hebbel once wrote, "Life is not anything; it is only the opportunity for something."

UNCONDITIONAL LOVE

Many people, especially cancer patients, grow up believing there is some terrible flaw at the center of their being, a defect they must hide if they are to have any chance for love. Feeling unlovable and condemned to loneliness if their true selves become known, such individuals set up defenses against sharing their innermost feelings with anyone. They feel their ability to love shriveling up, which leads to further despair. Dostoyevsky expressed the feeling when he wrote, "I am convinced that the only Hell which exists is the inability to love." Because such people feel a profound emptiness inside, they come to see all relationships and transactions in terms of *getting* something to fill the vaguely understood void within. They give love only on condition that they get something for it, whether comfort, security, praise, or a similar love. This "if" love is exhausting and prevents you from expressing your authentic self. It leads to an even deeper sense of emptiness, which keeps the vicious circle going.

I feel that all disease is ultimately related to a lack of love, or to love that is only conditional, for the exhaustion and depression of the immune system thus created leads to physical vulnerability. I also feel that all healing is related to the ability to give and accept unconditional love. This was strikingly borne out in the story of one of my cervical cancer patients, a secretary named Sherry.

As a child, Sherry felt unloved by her stepmother, and as a teenager she formed a strong attachment to one of her teachers. One day, in the school gym, Sherry told some of her friends that she loved Mrs. Johnson. Some of the children told the teacher, "Sherry loves you," and she called Sherry into her office.

"Sherry, do you love me from near or far?" Mrs. Johnson asked. The girl didn't know what the woman was talking about, so she said, "From near."

Mrs. Johnson then called Sherry's stepmother and told her that her daughter was a lesbian. When Sherry came home from school that day, her stepmother confronted her with the information. As she later told me, "I didn't know what 'lesbian' meant, but I got the message that love gets you in trouble, and I decided to stop loving."

Sherry lost her friends and became so lonely and desperate that she "would get dressed and walk the streets hoping people would look out their windows and wave at me." When she finally got married, she couldn't believe in her husband's love, and kept asking him, over and over, if he loved her. "I know if I hadn't developed cancer," she said, "he would have left me."

The impact of the disease, as well as group therapy in ECaP, enabled Sherry to change her outlook. She opened her heart to love, revitalized her marriage, and made a stand against her illness.

She was doing very well—and had even gone back to work —until her birthday. With six children, her husband, and her father-in-law all living in the same house, there was not one present for Sherry. Everybody had a reason, but underneath

they were all saying, "We're getting used to your being dead."
She hid her pain and despair from everyone, and two months
later she had a recurrence.

Once when I visited her soon afterward, she told me she
was "so upset about dying, because I'm trying to prove what
you're doing is right." She was still trying to stay alive for the
wrong reasons—to please other people instead of herself. And
all because of the lack of real love in her formative years. She
and her husband were never able to share their deepest feelings, though I kept trying to help them do so. Once I gave a
talk near Sherry's office and told them I'd dedicate it to her,
hoping the whole family would come. Her husband wrote me
a note saying, "I'm sorry, I'm busy that night, but call me if you
want to." However, the note had no name, address, or phone
number. Its unconscious message was, "Don't call me."

When I can get people to accept themselves as whole
individuals, lovable as they are, they become able to give from
an inner strength. They find that unconditional love does not
subtract from some limited emotional storehouse. Instead it
multiplies itself. It feels good to give, it makes the recipient
feel good, and sooner or later it returns. As Walt Whitman
wrote:

> Sometimes with one I love I fill myself with rage
>   for fear I effuse unreturned love,
> But now I think there is no unreturned love.
> The pay is certain, one way or another.
> (I loved a certain person ardently, and my love was
>   not returned,
> Yet out of that I have written these songs.)

One of the immediate rewards is a "live" message to the
body. I am convinced that unconditional love is the most powerful known stimulant of the immune system. If I told patients
to raise their blood levels of immune globulins or killer T cells,
no one would know how. But if I can teach them to love
themselves and others fully, the same changes happen automatically. The truth is: love heals.

I realized this intuitively many years ago, during my residency. A gentleman with severe staphylococcal pneumonia and empyema (an accumulation of pus in the chest) had gone into cardiac arrest. I gave him mouth-to-mouth resuscitation. When I came out of the room, the nurses were all shaking their heads and saying, "You're going to get sick. How could you do that?" I had a feeling then that my body would resist the infection because I had acted out of love for the man, and indeed I didn't get sick.

Years later I heard an account of a nearly identical experience by Dr. Jerry Jampolsky, of the Center for Attitudinal Healing in Tiburon, California. As part of his training, Jerry was sent to a tuberculosis sanatorium. He was frightened that he would contract the disease, and decided that he could take a deep breath when he got there, and hold it for three months. One night he was called to see a woman with active tuberculosis, who'd had a massive pulmonary hemorrhage and cardiac arrest. He gave her mouth-to-mouth resuscitation, and the nurses told him, "How could you do that? Now you're going to get tuberculosis." He never did, and he realized that he was not vulnerable while he was doing something for someone out of love. His realization strengthened mine, and now I've come to understand that this is why Mother Teresa and dedicated nurses can work among hundreds of sick, infected people every day without becoming ill. As the medieval German mystic Meister Eckhart wrote:

The bodily food we take is changed into us, but the spiritual food we receive changes us into itself; therefore divine love is not taken into us, for that would make two things. But divine love takes us into itself, and we are one with it.

SCIENCE AND THE HEALING SPIRIT

Even though love is hard to study scientifically, medical research is beginning to confirm its effects. At the Menninger Foundation in Topeka, Kansas, people who are *in* love, in the romantic sense, have been found to have reduced levels of lactic acid in their blood, making them less tired, and higher levels of endorphins, making them euphoric and less subject to pain. Their white blood cells also responded better when faced with infections, and thus they got fewer colds. Dr. Fred Cornhill and Murina Levesque of the Ohio State University College of Medicine reported in 1979 that "tender loving care" reduced atherosclerosis and the risk of heart attack by about 50 percent in rabbits fed large amounts of cholesterol. We also know that infants who do not receive love will waste away and die, even under the best conditions of sanitation and nutrition. The reason has been found by Dr. Christopher Coe of Stanford, who proved that the separation of infant monkeys from their mothers suppresses the babies' immune systems.

In 1982, Harvard psychologists David McClelland and Carol Kirshnit found that even movies about love increase levels of immunoglobulin-A in the saliva, the first line of defense against colds and other viral diseases. A Nazi propaganda film and a short on gardening had no effect, but a documentary on Mother Teresa's work produced a sharp rise in immunoglobulin—especially in persons motivated by altruism. However, the effect was unrelated to the subjects' conscious like or dislike of Mother Teresa, suggesting that the images of love had their effect at the unconscious level. Although the improvement lasted less than an hour, it could be prolonged by having the subjects think about times in their lives when they had been nurtured by someone.

Some of the most telling work has been done in Israel by Jack Medalie and Uri Goldbourt. The two researchers studied ten thousand men with the risk factors for angina pectoris—abnormal heart rhythms and high anxiety levels. Medalie and Goldbourt used psychological tests and questionnaires to find out what other factors determined which men would actually develop the chest pains. The most accurate predictor turned out to be a "No" answer to the question "Does your wife show you her love?" Furthermore, as Leo Buscaglia has pointed out, insurance companies have found that if a wife kisses her husband good-bye in the morning he has fewer auto accidents and lives five years longer.

Unfortunately, there isn't always a direct relationship between spiritual change or white-cell count and the cure of an illness. The idea is to love because it feels good, not because it will help us live forever. Love is the end itself, not the means. Love makes life worth living, no matter how long life lasts. It also increases the likelihood of physical healing, but that is the bonus, the icing on the cake.

Yet, though quality of life is the most important thing, people naturally want to extend its quantity, too. Most of the people who have changed in response to illness, those mentioned in these pages and thousands more like them, have outlived their doctors' expectations. By their own lives they have proven that love and authentic spirituality do increase one's time as well as one's joy. In the final analysis, this kind of evidence on the person-by-person level is the important kind. However, a small but growing handful of investigators are placing this most difficult of research subjects on a scientific basis. Their results, though preliminary, support what exceptional patients have learned.

The average survival time of the Simontons' patients is about two and a half times that of similar patients who receive only the standard medical treatments. About 10 percent of their patients remain disease-free past the standard five-year definition of a cancer cure—an extraordinarily high number compared with the rate of self-induced healing among seriously ill or "terminal" cancer patients in general. Yet this number should be even higher. These patients are self-selected, having traveled long distances for the program and put great energy into it. I believe that with more emphasis on spiritual growth and availability of therapy programs, there would be an even higher survival rate among these highly motivated patients.

Dr. Kenneth Pelletier has made a psychological study of many patients who recovered despite great odds. He found five characteristics common to all of them:

1. Profound intrapsychic change through meditation, prayer, or other spiritual practice.
2. Profound interpersonal changes, as a result: Their relations with other people had been placed on a more solid footing.

3. Alterations in diet: These people no longer took their food for granted. They chose their food carefully for optimum nutrition.
4. A deep sense of the spiritual as well as material aspects of life.
5. A feeling that their recovery was not a gift nor spontaneous remission, but rather a long, hard struggle that they had won for themselves.

In 1977 a research group led by Dr. Edward Gilbert of Denver's Presbyterian Medical Center completed one of the first controlled tests of psychological treatment of cancer patients. Gilbert and his co-workers asked independent physicians to examine a group of forty-eight patients and predict how long they could expect to live using standard medical treatments. The patients entered an eight-week program of individual and group therapy, biofeedback, and training in meditation and visualization. Then the patients were tested by independent psychiatrists to see which ones had made the most positive changes in their lives. Five patients were graded as having changed most significantly, and four of these far exceeded medical expectations. Of the other twenty-five then remaining in the group, only one outlived the initial prognosis by a similar margin.

One statistical study has been attempted with breast cancer patients in ECaP by medical student George Gellert and Yale epidemiologist Hal Morgenstern. It showed an average survival time strikingly greater during the follow up period, than that of members of a comparison group. However, a significant number of ECaP members had already exceeded predictions before joining the group, so there is a self-selection process at work that is hard to keep from skewing the results. At the end of Morgenstern's study, he noted that new patients entering ECaP do begin to show a higher survival rate and that this deserves careful observation and follow-up, which we are now planning.

It isn't easy to put love under a microscope, and because I'm a practicing physician trying to help people here and now, I prefer to deal with individuals and effective techniques, and let others take care of the statistics. There is also a lack of grant money for this research, but that will surely change as psychoneuroimmunology becomes more widely accepted. Research gradually improves medical care, and I believe that someday we will understand the physiological and psychological workings of love well enough to turn on its full force more reliably. Once it is scientific, it will be accepted.

When doctors and patients understand the healing power of love, we will begin to add another dimension to medicine. Then we will be well on our way to the glorious revelation predicted by Teilhard de Chardin in these famous words:

Someday, after we have mastered the winds, the waves, the tides and gravity, we shall harness for God the energies of love. Then for the second time in the history of the world, man will have discovered fire.

EMOTIONAL SUPPORT

We encourage spouses, relatives, and friends of patients to attend ECaP meetings, because it's much harder for one person to change while loved ones continue in the old patterns. Ideally, the entire family or extended family should be treated as a unit. We have to understand that, in a sense, *everyone* has the disease when it strikes one family member. In a group setting, we can often help people see how destructive behavior patterns interact to reinforce each other, and how love heals.

It's also well known that a focus outside the self helps people survive a crisis. London sociologist George W. Brown reported in 1975 that, based on psychiatric testing, "an intimate and confiding (but not necessarily sexual) relationship with a husband or boyfriend" reduced the likelihood of depression among women who had recently undergone severe stress of any kind. In 1979 L. F. Berkman and S. L. Syme reported long-term work with 4,725 adults in Alameda County, California. They studied the effects of marriage, church and club memberships, and friends, with controls for smoking, obesity, and other previous health problems. The researchers found that those with the fewest social contacts had a death rate two and a half times higher than those who had the most social contacts. Those who have pets live longer after heart attacks than those who don't, and nearly everyone knows someone who has postponed death until after Christmas, a reunion, or a birthday.

Love of other people always is a sustaining factor. In a sense, however, living *for* others is a "gimmick," a stopgap measure like surgery or chemotherapy, which can buy time until people learn to live authentically for themselves.

We all know that one of our basic needs is someone in whom to confide, and recent research is proving that confession is good for the body as well as the soul. Several statistical studies have shown that people in psychotherapy visit physicians less often than people not in therapy.

In experiments spanning the early 1980s, James Pennebaker, a psychologist at Southern Methodist University, has shown that sharing sorrow with someone else protects people from the stress of loss. Pennebaker studied men and women whose spouses had committed suicide or died in auto accidents and found that those who bore their grief alone had a much higher than average rate of illness, while those who could talk over their troubles with someone else had no increase in health problems. In another experiment, Pennebaker told volunteers he would ask them to talk about a traumatic event in their lives, either into a tape recorder or in a simulated confessional booth. When he had them describe some trivial event instead, physiological measurements showed them to be tense, but when later they were asked to reveal the tragedy after all, their bodies relaxed completely, even though many cried and expressed powerful emotions.

Writing apparently works, too. Students who wrote about their traumas made fewer visits to physicians in the ensuing six months than did others who wrote about less important subjects. Keeping a diary gets us in touch with our thoughts. It's really a type of meditation. When I suggest keeping a diary, I don't mean where you went that day, but what you thought that day. It makes us aware how active our minds are while we're paying no attention to our thoughts, as we shower or eat.

A diary can help us become conscious of all these ideas and learn from them.

The people in a patient's emotional support network often need to be educated, too. Many people simply don't know how to relate to someone who has a life-threatening illness. The only essential, really, is an honest optimism. Patients need people to help them keep sight of their hopes and the joys that are possible as long as life goes on. But patients sometimes need to gently remind friends and loved ones that a false determination to be constantly upbeat, no matter what the situation, is destructive. It springs from the fears of disability and death that illness evokes in those who are well. It's a natural reaction, but it must be faced, and it's one area where group sessions can be enormously helpful. Beyhan Lowman, who died of cancer at thirty-one in 1978, left behind *A Spirit Soars*, a booklet that serves as a marvelous guide to those facing the same challenge. In it she wrote poignantly of the patient's need for honesty:

Although everyone around me was trying his best to be light-hearted and optimistic, somehow the effect on me was just the opposite. Suddenly being thrust into a situation where everyone behaved only positively while around me made me realize to what extent I was no longer part of that world.

The doctors and nurses who cared for me could not always have a good day. They must have been tired of turning me over in bed or hearing me complain. But, I never saw that. The lab technician taking a blood sample must have been frustrated because my veins were so hard to find. But, she always smiled through gritted teeth. Many times I heard the medical staff outside my door talking in agitated tones. But then, they always appeared in my room as if they were actors going onstage in a well-rehearsed role.

The same was true of my family and friends. Everyone tried to help by telling me how wonderful and courageous I was. Even the man in my life treated me differently. I knew he must have felt some sense of injustice at being involved with a dying woman —a development he never bargained for. Yet, he never expressed it to me. Of course, his intentions were to protect me, but I would have had a lot to say to him. Instead of probing his emotions, which would have included me in the life process, I allowed myself to feel excluded by his silence.

Since disease has usually fulfilled some psychological need for the patient, it's also important to encourage change by doing things that reward health, not continued illness. As adapted from a list given by the Simontons, these include:

1. Encourage the patient to be active and do things for himself.
2. Comment when the patient improves. Don't get so involved with difficulties that you can't see anything except signs of disease.
3. Spend time in activities unrelated to the illness.
4. Continue the relationship at its new and deeper level as the patient recovers.

It's equally important for couples to continue some form of physical intimacy through illness. Like many of the elderly, severely ill patients often suffer from "skin starvation," a literal separation from life, when touching stops. If lovemaking becomes difficult, there are usually alternative ways of sexual gratification possible within a couple's values, ingenuity, and physical condition. Caresses, hugs, kisses, and hand holding are *always* possible. One of my patients had marked ascites (abdominal distention), which was uncomfortable if her husband pushed against it. So she devised a way in which they could kiss, touch shoulders and knees, and avoid pressure on her abdomen.

I find that the resumption of loving—by touching and caressing, not necessarily sexual activity—after surgery or illness is a crucial sign of marital support for a full recovery, especially after operations such as mastectomy. Spouses often need counseling to adapt to such changes in their lovers' bodies, and this is another problem for which groups like ECaP are invaluable. When a couple can survive such hardship, each knows ever afterward that they have an unshakable foundation on which to build the rest of their lives. Richard Selzer wrote eloquently of this bond in an essay called "Lessons from the Art of Surgery":

> The young woman speaks. "Will my mouth always be like this?" she asks.
> "Yes," I say, "it will. It is because the nerve was cut."
> She nods, and is silent. But the young man smiles.
> "I like it," he says. "It is kind of cute."
> All at once I *know* who he is. I understand, and I lower my gaze. One is not bold in an encounter with a god. Unmindful, he bends to kiss her crooked mouth, and I so close I can see how he twists his own lips to accommodate to hers, to show her that their kiss still works. I remember that the gods appeared in ancient Greece as mortals, and I hold my breath and let the wonder in.

There's something more that patients need from their loved ones, perhaps the most difficult requirement of all—the need to deal with fears and long-standing resentments or conflicts, the "unfinished business," as Elisabeth Kübler-Ross calls it. This comes about through the same two linked opposites we've been discussing in various ways throughout this chapter —self-love *and* love for others, assertiveness *and* forgiveness.

TRANSCENDING FEAR

To unblock the fountain of love and enter on the path of creative, spiritual growth, we must let go of our fears ("leave our troubles to God"). But this is very hard, particularly when it looks as though we're *not* going to die tomorrow. When we don't have that time limit, it's often harder to let go. To accomplish this "simple" change, we must work through our negative emotions and transcend them. This is impossible until we realize that no one *makes* us happy or sad. Our emotions don't *happen* to us so much as we *choose* them. In fact, our own thoughts, emotions, and actions are the only things we really do control. In the first century A.D., the Greek thinker Epictetus made this fact the foundation of his philosophy, declaring that all unhappiness arises from attempts to control events and other people, over which one has no power. The same futile attempt, born of our fears and resentments, weakens the body and leads to disease.

At one level there is nothing to fear but, obviously, this can be taken too literally and seriously. For example, fear is natural in life-threatening situations—such as in high places and near loud noises—but every other fear is abnormal. We will never meet anything we can't handle. I know this by definition because no patient ever wants to exchange diseases. We each are more comfortable with our own problems. I have a list of positive sayings above our kitchen table. Our young daughter Carolyn helped teach me the futility of getting caught up in words. In the middle of a dinner-table argument among our children, I asked everyone, "Do you want peace or do you want conflict?" The first item on the list. Our daughter, who has a mild hearing loss, answered, "I'll have pizza." We all laughed, and the argument stopped. The aim here is not to lay down strict rules of behavior but rather to use the imperfect medium of words to point toward a new psychological reality —a happiness we can choose, independent of external conditions.

A positive outlook can be cultivated as can a negative one be inculcated by a lifetime of conditioning. In fact, psychologists long ago discovered that emotions can be modified merely by adopting the facial expression of a contrary emotion. Recently Dr. Paul Ekman of the University of California at San Francisco distinguished eighteen anatomically different types of smiles. He found that persons trained to control individual facial muscles voluntarily could affect physiological measurements of emotion by assuming the facial position of a particular smile.

Sadness can be lessened by looking in the mirror and smiling, as long as one is not denying the sadness. Performing will not work, but truly putting on a smile will create a different message that is fed back into the nervous system. You can grieve for a loss, yet still keep yourself from losing all perspective, all appreciation for the good things that remain in your life.

Scientists who have studied responses to stress have found that ineffectual anger is the emotion most destructive to homeostasis. A serene acceptance of *what is* promotes health, but by keeping the mind clear it also puts a person in a better position to change things that need changing. Hence, as Dr. Wallace Ellerbroek has written, we should "be keeping pleasant thoughts in our heads as well as pleasant expressions on our faces, and behaving in general as if we were not going to our own funerals."

It is necessary for those dealing with illness to reaffirm themselves constantly with positive messages. A patient needs to stop getting up every day saying, "I have cancer. I'm too weak or depressed to do anything," and start saying instead, "Today can be beautiful. Today can be different *because* of the cancer." The disease can be a motivator for change. As Lois Becker wrote in her letter to me,

I think of cancer every day, but I also think of how strong my body is, how good it feels most of the time. I still talk to my insides. I have a feeling of integration of body, mind and, probably, spirit, which I never before experienced.

Letting go of fear is the sticking point for many people. It's easier if you see every interchange as either a request for or a giving of love. A frightened person is really saying, "Love me." But we tend to reject that person and get angry. Then he or she gets more frightened and often hoards anger until it hardens into resentment or hate. *To hate is easy, but it is healthier to love.* When you're feeling afraid, if you ask someone for a hug, for some love, the fear will quiet down.

One night I was in the emergency room to examine a patient, and a man wandered out of the psychiatric wing. He walked straight toward me—because of my shaved head, I believe—and started berating me, screaming about my ancestors and sexual habits. Everyone else disappeared into the woodwork except the patients sitting up in their cubicles watching. As he stood there screaming at me, I knew I had to see my patient, and I wondered how I was going to take care of this situation. I thought about all my sermons, and I looked him in the eye and said, "I love you." He stopped as if he'd been hit in the head with a mallet. He turned around and went quietly back into his room and sat down. The chief of nursing in the emergency room said, "You handled that beautifully." And I said, "Thanks for your help."

Love is incredibly powerful in the midst of conflict. In most families I have no trouble getting people to say, "I hate you." "I love you" is much harder. Patients often must say it by letter or phone before they can say it face to face—because it's the "I love you" that carries the real emotional power.

There really isn't anything you can't handle. *I* know that, even though you may not know it yet. Someone may tell me, "I'm frightened. My husband has run off with another woman. I have cancer now, and I've got five kids at home. I don't know what to do." From experience with other patients I can now tell that person, "You know what's going to happen a year from now? You'll ask me, 'Do you know anyone else with a similar problem? I'll call them up and offer my help.' " You *are* strong enough to get through all those things.

I know a woman named Emily who was so fearful she wouldn't go out in the *rain*. She wouldn't sign checks, either. She avoided almost all of life's joys and responsibilities. Her husband finally left her, and you couldn't blame him. Then she developed leukemia and went through an incredible metamorphosis. When last seen, she was at a political rally, yelling at the top of her lungs. Her husband would remarry the woman she has become. But it took leukemia to get her to wake up and live. For many people, it takes the knowledge that we won't live forever—so why be afraid to love?

TRANSCENDING HATE

Resentments and hate are the obstacles that keep many people from clearing up their unfinished emotional business and achieving harmony with others. Transcending fear opens the way to forgiveness of those who have wronged you, and it releases a love that can make you psychologically immune to your environment. Choosing to love and hold on to the meaning of life increases the chances of survival under *all* conditions. Psychiatrist Viktor Frankl, a survivor of the Nazi death camps, wrote in his memoir *Man's Search for Meaning* that the guards found it easier to kill those who seemed ready to die than those who looked at their captors, with a spark of life in their eyes. Love saved Frankl's life at one point. When he and his fellow prisoners were told that a train was going to a work camp where conditions would be better, he gave his place to someone else. The train went to one of the gas chambers.

Another survivor, Jack Schwarz, has told how he passed out during a whipping and had a vision of Christ. Filled with love from the image, he said to his torturer, "Ich liebe dich." The guard was so shocked that he stopped, and he was even more astounded when he saw right before his eyes the prisoner's wounds healing within moments.

Psychiatrist George Ritchie, author of *Return from Tomorrow,* tells this story of "Wild Bill," one of the death-camp survivors with whom he worked after the liberation:

["Wild Bill"] was one of the inmates of the concentration camp, but obviously he hadn't been there long: His posture was erect, his eyes bright, his energy indefatigable. Since he was fluent in English, French, German and Russian, as well as Polish, he became a kind of unofficial camp translator. . . .

Though Wild Bill worked fifteen and sixteen hours a day, he showed no signs of weariness. While the rest of us were drooping with fatigue, he seemed to gain strength. . . .

I was astonished to learn when Wild Bill's own papers came before us one day, that he had been in Wuppertal since 1939! For six years he had lived on the same starvation diet, slept in the same airless and disease-ridden barracks as everyone else, but without the least physical or mental deterioration. . . .

Wild Bill was our greatest asset, reasoning with the different groups, counseling forgiveness.

"It's not easy for some of them to forgive," I commented to him one day. . . . "So many of them have lost members of their families."

"We lived in the Jewish section of Warsaw," he began slowly, the first words I had heard him speak about himself, "my wife, our two daughters, and our three little boys. When the Germans reached our street they lined everyone against a wall and opened up with machine guns. I begged to be allowed to die with my family, but because I spoke German they put me in a work group."

"I had to decide right then," he continued, "whether to let myself hate the soldiers who had done this. It was an easy decision, really. I was a lawyer. In my practice I had seen too often what hate could do to people's minds and bodies. Hate had just killed the six people who mattered most to me in the world. I decided then that I would spend the rest of my life—whether it was a few days or many years—loving every person I came in contact with." This was the power that had kept a man well in the face of every privation.

I'm not saying all the survivors came through by being able to love the Nazis as human beings, and I'm certainly not saying everybody else died because they didn't love enough. Many hung on to life so they could be witnesses to the world. Some did it by turning "hatred into energy," which was the slogan that enabled the Vietnamese to survive forty years of war and overcome the Japanese, French, and Americans—but you have to be careful that you don't end up becoming like your enemies. To attempt Wild Bill's kind of love just because somebody says it's righteous would be a pathetic hypocrisy. Such love may have little to do with the individuals in the drama but rather may be a welling forth of a universal power —God or the basic goodness of humanity—through the deepest wounds of the spirit.

What I am saying is that love can save *you!* You can look at a murderer with love based on the fact that you know what got him where he is. I'm not suggesting you love atrocities, but even the most depraved person started out as an innocent baby. We have to remember that all of us are created by our parents and society. If we get the wrong messages from them and receive no love from them, then any of us can end up a Hitler. This is not an acceptance of evil, but rather a refusal to sink to its level. As Martin Luther King, Sr., has said, "Hate won't bring my family back." You may not be able to change your oppressor or save your life by your love, but you can keep hatred from destroying *your* heart, mind, and life, as it has destroyed his.

Among my patients I meet many who are dealing with "impossible" spouses. There are two ways out: You can either divorce your "Hitler" or stay and try to change him or her with love. I remember a woman named Ruth, who once told me, "I'll make this marriage work if it kills me." She developed extensive metastatic breast cancer and became so depressed that she was considering suicide. Then one day Ruth was in the audience at one of my talks. The subject of suicide came up, and a young woman in the audience related how her father had killed himself and her life had been devastated, both because of the loss itself and because she couldn't deal with her father's lack of courage. Her story moved Ruth so much that she found new courage within herself, decided to live, and left her husband.

However, when you realize that both you and your "Hitler" are only human, you can probably learn to live together, helping each other change. Nothing helps someone become better as much as someone else granting the possibility. As Goethe wrote, "If you treat an individual as he is, he will stay that way, but if you treat him as if he were what he could be, he will become what he could be." I find it useful to remember what Martin Luther King, Jr., once wrote about Jesus' command to love your enemies:

Forgiveness does not mean ignoring what has been done or putting a false label on an evil act. It means, rather, that the evil act no longer remains as a barrier to the relationship. . . . We must recognize that the evil deed of the enemy neighbor, the thing that hurts, never quite expresses all that he is. An element of goodness may be found even in our worst enemy.

The meaning of love is not to be confused with some sentimental outpouring. Love is something much deeper than emotional bosh. . . . Now we can see what Jesus meant when he said, "Love your enemies." We should be happy that he did not say, "Like your enemies." It is almost impossible to like some people. "Like" is a sentimental and affectionate word. How can we be affectionate toward a person whose avowed aim is to crush our very being and place innumerable stumbling blocks in our path? How can we like a person who is threatening our children or bombing our homes? That is impossible. But Jesus recognized that *love* is greater than *like*. When Jesus bids us to love our enemies, he is speaking of understanding and creative, redemptive goodwill for all men. Only by following this way and responding with this type of love are we able to be children of our Father who is in heaven.

The real test is not whether we could be crucified to save mankind but whether we can live with someone who snores.

You have to remember that you cannot change anyone. You can only change yourself. But remember you create the other person by what you're like. This often gives a wife, for example, great power. Eleanor, one of my patients, works with her husband in real estate. She's capable of making million-dollar deals, but he criticizes the way she dresses, even sends her back in the house to change her clothes when they're ready to go out to dinner. I said, "Okay, then tell him you can't make decisions. Don't wash, clean, cook, keep the books, or do any of the other things he expects of you. If he asks, 'Where's dinner?' tell him you couldn't decide what to buy at the supermarket. Tell him you couldn't decide what detergent to buy, so the laundry isn't done. Tell him how indecisive you are, and he'll have to take over everything. Then he'll realize how much you do, and what you're capable of."

Taking care of unfinished business may someday come to be recognized as the most effective pain reliever and preparation for surgery. I recall a medical student named Karen who visited ECaP after she'd learned her boyfriend's father was to undergo surgery for lung cancer. She'd spent a busy week checking to make sure the surgeon was well qualified. Then, on the way to the hospital, she remembered something I often ask group members: she asked her boyfriend what he would say to his father if he knew his father were going to die tomorrow.

In the hospital, the young man went up to his father, who had been an alcoholic, and said, "Dad, there were times you beat me, locked me in the trunk of the car, and did other things

to me, but I want you to know I love you and forgive you."
They embraced and cried.

Naturally, the father came through surgery without difficulty. When Karen came to her next meeting, she told us what
happened and said, "It wasn't so important to spend all that
energy checking the surgeon's credentials. What was important was saying 'I love you.'"

When speaking at workshops I often ask, "If you knew you
were going to die on the way home, would you need to use the
phone?" If the answer is yes, I say, "Okay, if you promise when
you get home to pick up the phone and make all those calls,
I'll guarantee a safe trip home."

When you suffer a misfortune, you are faced with the
choice of what to do with it. You can wring good from it, or
more pain. Out of the ordeal of his son's death, Rabbi Kushner
was eventually able to write a book, *When Bad Things Happen
to Good People*, which has helped thousands of people through
similar tragedies. In that way, the life that has been lost is given
meaning through what is created out of the pain.

The ability to see something good in adversity is perhaps
the central trait needed by patients. As Viktor Frankl has written: "To live is to suffer; to survive is to find meaning in the
suffering." Death or the threat of death has been called the
ultimate teacher, for it goads us into appreciating to the utmost
what we have or can do today.

My wife and I had to learn this lesson during a week in
which we thought our son Keith, at the age of eight, had a
malignant bone tumor. He told me he had a pain in his leg. At
first I said he should take hot baths as any good doctor would
suggest. Then one day, while I was lacing his ice skates, he told
me the pain wasn't going away, and he suggested an x-ray. My
thought was that we'll teach him a lesson. He'll probably have
a superficial break in the bone, and then he'll be sorry he got
the x-ray—he'll have to wear a cast for a fracture that would
have healed without one. Instead, the x-ray showed a lytic
bone lesion. According to all my medical books this represented a malignancy, and our beautiful child would be dead
within a year. The five days before he was admitted to the
hospital for surgery were a horror and my guilt added to this,

a guilt all parents feel. It was impossible to think, love, concentrate, or talk. Fortunately, the tumor proved benign and was removed easily with a small portion of the bone.

However, the experience was one of our most important lessons. It showed us what patients and their families must deal with. Moreover, it taught my wife and me about survival. Our daughter Carolyn said to me one day at breakfast, "Dad, do you ever think who will die first?" I said, "That is not the issue. The issue is that the rest of us will go on living and giving more to the world to make the life of the one who died more meaningful."

Unfortunately, most of us must suffer before we can be transformed. My wife, Bobbie, and I were sitting in the kitchen when the garbage disposal jammed. I said, "What shall I do?" She said, "Just push the reset button." So I went to God and asked, "If you're such a great creator, why didn't you give us a reset button?" God answered, "I did give you a reset button, Bernie. It's called pain and suffering." It is only through pain that we change. It can be difficult to see our loved ones hurting but not changing. Our job is to love them. It is their pain that changes them, not our sermon.

Finding the ability to love requires giving up the fear, anguish, and despair that many people nurture. Many people have a lifetime of unresolved angers circulating through their minds and causing new stress with each recall. Confronting them and letting go of them involves honestly facing your own part in the problem, and forgiving yourself as well as the others you've resented and feared. If you do not forgive, you become like your enemy.

The children with whom Jerry Jampolsky works have expressed the lesson of transcendence superbly in the conclusion of a book they wrote together, called *There Is a Rainbow Behind Every Dark Cloud:*

> In summary, we think that your mind can do anything. You can learn to control your mind and decide to be happy "inside" with a smiling heart, in spite of what happens to you on the "outside."
> Whether you are sick or well, when you give help and love

to others, it makes you feel warm and peaceful inside. We learned that, when you give love, you receive it at the same time.

And letting go of the past and forgiving everyone and everything sure helps you not be afraid.

Remember that you are love. So let your love expand, and love yourself and everyone. When you love and really feel joined with everyone, everything, and with God, you can feel happy and safe inside.

And don't forget, when you have total Faith that we are always connected to each other in love, you will surely find a rainbow on the other side of any dark cloud.

The phenomenal energy that can be liberated by surrendering our negative emotions was described to me in a letter from Denise, a breast-cancer patient who visited the congregation of a faith healer in Worcester, Massachusetts. She wrote:

After his sermon, he said that each one would know in their heart if they were the one to be called. He turned around to his audience of over 1500 people and said, "I have a strong experience with someone concerning a rose. She has a disease in her chest area." I felt my insides move as I recalled the night before while I was at dinner, when I took a fresh rose out of the vase on our table, and smelled it. Someone had told me I had to take time to smell the flowers of life. However, I didn't stand up. I thought it couldn't be me.

The healer then approached a woman who had stood up. Her name was Rose, and she had breast cancer. He blessed her but said, "You are not the one I am experiencing."

He said, "She also has breast cancer, and is wearing a beige top." That morning I had put on a pair of black slacks and a long-sleeved black blouse. Then I decided to put on my short-sleeved beige blouse as an overlay, felt too fat, and took it off, and then decided to put it back on again.

At this point I stood up, and he called me down to the front of the audience. He asked me about my illness, and as I stood there full of tears and emotions, I shall never forget how his face looked. He didn't have any eyes, just dark pools of infinity. As he anointed my forehead, he said, *"You have to let go of your anguish."* And with this, I experienced a bolt of energy that passed through my body. I felt a scream come from my mouth, and I fell toward the floor into the arms of the ushers behind me.

This experience was a turning point for Denise. She began to be able to set priorities for herself and make choices based on her own needs. She used psychotherapy and chemotherapy, ended a relationship she felt to be damaging to her, and sold her business, which had been a major source of stress. Finally allowing herself to express a lifetime of pent-up anger, frustration, and sadness, she cried for days, and found that for the first time she was able to accept the child within her. At the end of her letter, she wrote, "This was the first time I had ever given myself the privilege and dignity to mourn my own pains and agonies. Now that all the debris has moved from my soul, my [inner] child and I are one. I feel total integration, self love, and forgiveness. I need never judge others, for I no longer need to judge myself."

Spirituality, unconditional love, and the ability to see that pain and problems are opportunities for growth and redirection—these things allow us to make the best of the time we have. Then we realize that the present moment is all we have, but it is infinite. We see that there is no real past or future, and that as soon as we start thinking in terms of past and future—regretting and wishing—we lose ourselves in judgemental thinking. In one of the countries where people regularly live to be a hundred, people have a saying: "Yesterday is gone, tomorrow isn't here yet, so what is there to worry about?"

Many people are able to let go of their fears and resentments only when they are nearly dead. Several years ago Dr. Ellerbroek described one such case in the following terms:

Her pelvis, bladder and rectum had been removed—until she seemed to be nothing more than a bag of flesh draped over a skeleton that offered shelter not for internal organs but for spreading tumors. She asked to be allowed to die on the shore of a local lake. In those peaceful surroundings, something happened; she jettisoned her anger and depression, her spirit, like a balloon freed of useless weight, soared—and her tumors started to shrink. She was cured.

Later Ellerbroek reflected on this and similar cases with these words:

It is my primary belief that we were sold a big bill of goods when we were little. We were taught that under certain circumstances it is appropriate to be angry, and that under all circumstances it is appropriate to be depressed. I'm here to say that in my own personal, solitary opinion—and totally contrary to the beliefs of almost all the psychiatrists I know—I believe that anger and depression are pathological emotions, that they are immediately responsible for the vast majority of human ills, including cancer. I have collected 57 extremely well documented so-called cancer miracles. A cancer miracle is when a person didn't die when they absolutely, positively were supposed to. At a certain particular moment in time they decided that the anger and the depression were probably not the best way to go, since they had such a little bit of time left, and so they went from that to being loving, caring, no longer angry, no longer depressed, and able to talk to the people they loved. These 57 people had the same pattern. They gave up, totally, their anger, and they gave up, totally, their depression, by specifically a decision to do so. And at that point the tumors started to shrink.

(I use the word "resentment" instead of "anger," because I think anger is a normal emotion if it is expressed when felt. Then it is over with. If one keeps a lid on it, it develops into resentment or hate. Sooner or later, resentment and hate explode, destroying others, or they are held in, destroying oneself.)

The transcendence described by Ellerbroek is precisely the essence of the religious experience as it was described by Jung in *Psychology and Religion:*

They came to themselves, they could accept themselves, they were able to become reconciled to themselves and by this they were also reconciled to adverse circumstances and events. This is much like what was formerly expressed by saying: He has made his peace with God, he has sacrificed his own will, he has submitted himself to the will of God.

To those rationalists who argue that any such experience is a self-delusion, Jung adds an especially apt reply:

Is there any better truth about ultimate things than the one that helps you to live? This is the reason why I take carefully into account the symbols produced by the unconscious mind. They are the only things able to convince the critical mind of modern people. They are convincing for very old-fashioned reasons. They are simply overwhelming, which is an English rendering of the Latin word "convincere." The thing that cures a neurosis must be as convincing as the neurosis; and since the latter is only too real, the helpful experience must be of equal reality. It must be a very real illusion, if you want to put it pessimistically. But what is the difference between a real illusion and a healing religious experience? It is merely a difference in words. You can say, for instance, that life is a disease with a very bad prognosis, it lingers on for years to end with death; or that normality is a generally prevailing constitutional defect; or that man is an animal with a fatally overgrown brain. This kind of thinking is the prerogative of habitual grumblers with bad digestions. Nobody can know what the ultimate things are. We must, therefore, take them as we experience them. And if such experience helps to make your life healthier, more beautiful, more complete and more satisfactory to yourself and to those you love, you may safely say: "This was the grace of God."

Ellerbroek has concluded that patients with far advanced cancer must be near death before the turnaround can happen, but I know from my experience that people can change at any time. The earlier it occurs in the course of a disease, the greater the chances of recovery. If a person takes the spiritual path before becoming sick, he or she becomes practically invulnerable to disease and misfortune—at least in the psychological sense, and very often in the physical sense. As Norman Cousins wrote after his self-cure of ankylosing spondylitis, "I have learned never to underestimate the capacity of the human mind and body to regenerate, even when the prospects seem most wretched."

Dr. Granger Westberg, founder of numerous Wholistic Health Care Centers, in which doctors, nurses, and ministers work as a team, believes that the illnesses of about half to three-fourths of all patients originate in problems of the spirit rather than in breakdowns of the body. As he phrases it, the physical symptoms are often only the "tickets of admission" to a process of self-discovery and spiritual change. To begin that true healing, each of us must make the leap of faith described by French poet Guillaume Apollinaire, who once wrote:

Come to the edge.
No, we will fall.

Come to the edge.
No, we will fall.

They came to the edge.
He pushed them, and they flew.

9

*There is no difficulty that enough love will not
conquer; no disease that enough love will not heal; no
door that enough love will not open; no gulf that
enough love will not bridge; no wall that enough love
will not throw down; no sin that enough love will not
redeem. . . .
It makes no difference how deeply seated may be
the trouble; how hopeless the outlook; how muddled
the tangle; how great the mistake. A sufficient
realization of love will dissolve it all. If only you could
love enough you would be the happiest and most
powerful being in the world. . . .*

—EMMET FOX, The Sermon on the Mount

Love and Death

Five days before William Saroyan died in 1981, he called the
Associated Press to leave this statement: "Everybody has got
to die, but I have always believed an exception would be made
in my case. Now what?" His humor showed how alive one can
be even in the face of death.

Neal was a patient who had originally been diagnosed as
having carcinoma of the pancreas. He'd been told by his oncologist that he might live for a year or two. He exceeded that
expectation, only to find out years later, after a second biopsy,
that he had lymphoma instead of pancreatic cancer. He was
then told he might live many more years. Since he and the
family had been planning for his death, this news upset him.
As bizarre as it may sound, he called me at this time, telling
me how upset he was that the doctors said he might live a long
time. I said to him, "You know how doctors are. They're not
always right, you could die soon." He said, "You know, I can
always count on you to cheer me up." I allowed him to change
slowly. Within a few months he had readjusted to living.

Several years later Neal was taken to the emergency room

with a high fever. He had an out-of-body experience and was up above, looking down on the resuscitation. He heard the doctor say, "We'd better get his wife, because he's not going to make it." He was up above, thinking, "Don't bother my wife. I'll make it." And he did.

Some time later Neal asked to be admitted to the hospital. Having fought lymphoma valiantly for years, he was exhausted and ready to die. His wife worked in the hospital's medical library, and could be near him. It was extremely hard to convince the nurses that he was there to die. They would come in every day and say, "Finish your lunch. Eat everything on your plate." It took them awhile to shift gears and allow him to do what he felt was appropriate.

One day, with tears in his eyes, he called the nurses in and asked them to get his wife. He told her, "Honey, I've been there. It's warm and colorful and beautiful, and they said, 'It's your time.' But I said, 'No, I haven't said good-bye to my wife yet.' They said, 'But it's your time,' but I argued and kept saying, 'I haven't said good-bye.' Finally they said it was all right," and that was when he returned to the room and called the nurses. Neal and his wife said their good-byes, and he died quietly within twenty-four hours.

DYING AT PEACE

Exceptional patients have taught me that we have an amazing amount of control over our dying. Even a large-scale statistical study of several thousand deaths recently showed that nearly half came in the three months after birthdays, while only 8 percent occurred in the preceding quarter. I'm not saying that we can live as long as we want, but we don't have to die until we are ready. The most obvious proof of this is the time people die in the hospital. The vast majority die in the early hours of the morning when the lifesavers are resting and the family has left or fallen asleep. Then there is no interference with, or guilt over, leaving. All of us, especially those who are living with serious illness or trauma, are constantly balancing the rewards of life versus the "cost of living." One patient told me that as long as she had five good minutes a day she would keep on living. The pain and fear of dying come primarily from conflict, unfinished business, and hanging on so as not to "fail" one's family. We can learn to live each day as a unit—doing what needs to be done, giving and receiving love —and thus always being prepared to die. As one patient told me, "Death is not the worst thing. Life without love is far worse." Having mastered the art of living day by day, we can always manage twenty-four hours if we have an important goal to reach.

This postponement can last a long time. I was giving a pep talk on this subject to Melanie, a nurse with breast cancer. She said, "You don't have to tell me that. My mother came home one day when I was sixteen and said, 'Girls, I've been told I have leukemia and that I'm going to die within a year. But I'm not going to die until you're all married and out of the house.' " Eight years later she attended her youngest daughter's wedding.

Many times I have witnessed the death of people who have learned to love fully. It's a peaceful, pain-free letting-go, in which no time is spent dying. However, two conditions have to be met before this can happen: the doctor as lifesaver must be told when to stop, and loved ones must give the patient permission to go. They must share their love and grief, but let the dying person know that they will be able to survive. In other words, the dying person must not receive a "Don't die" message from the family. He or she must receive their love and support, and the knowledge that the loved ones will survive because they have been loved. The example the dying person has been reveals how precious life is, even as it is being given up.

Today I see that even death can be a form of healing. When patients whose bodies are tired and sore are at peace with themselves and their loved ones, they can choose death as their next treatment. They do not have pain because there is no conflict in their lives. They are at peace and comfortable. Often at that time they have a "little miracle" and go on living for a while, because there is so much peace that some healing does occur. But when they die they are *choosing* to leave their bodies because they can't use them for loving anymore. My own father told me about his grandfather, who at the age of ninety-one said, "Get my friends together and get me a bottle of schnapps. I'm going to die tonight." To humor him, the family complied. That night after the party he went upstairs, lay down, and died.

Each of us has that option. I might choose to live when someone else might choose to die, but that depends on what we need to accomplish and how much loving remains to be done. Death is no longer a failure but a natural option, and, since I have redefined myself as a healer and teacher, I can participate in this choice and help patients to keep on *living* until they die. We must realize people are not living or dying but alive or dead. Label someone terminal and he is treated as dead. This is wrong; if you are alive you can still participate by loving, laughing and living. Before I would accept a quadriplegic's decision to die I would have him take one month of art lessons from another quadriplegic who does incredibly beautiful paintings holding the brush in his mouth.

An elderly gentleman had fallen down the stairs and was admitted to the hospital in a coma. He and his wife had been married over sixty years. The next day she had a heart attack and was admitted to the medical service. He was in coma, she was on a respirator, and they were on two different floors. I suggested to the intern that he should let each of them know about the other's condition, since there obviously could be no direct communication. I said, "If one dies, the other ought to know what has happened." The interns all thought it was spooky, so I whispered in the ear of each what had happened to the other.

The next day I came to the hospital, and the intern said, "Do you know what happened?" I said, "No. What?" He said, "Mr. Smith died, and I had picked up the phone to call the intern on the medical floor to get the phone number of the niece who was the next of kin. The intern there said, 'That's funny. I'm looking for it. What do you need it for?' Mr. Smith had just died, and the other intern said his wife had just died. The wife followed him by five minutes." What a gentleman—he went and picked up his wife, and they left together.

A drawn-out, living death happens when feelings are unspoken, conflicts remain unresolved, and life goes on only for the sake of others. It occurs when the dying one receives "Don't die" messages, which define death as a failure, something that must be done in secret when doctors and loved ones are absent.

When people achieve peace with themselves and others, it becomes all right to die, to "relax and enjoy it," as one of my patients put it. But paradoxically, as Dr. Ellerbroek has found, this very acceptance may produce healing. I felt Valerie was only about forty-eight hours from death, and because of her husband's reluctance to accept the situation, I decided to help get the family together. On Tuesday night I explained the situation to her husband and suggested that he call their girls to come home from college. He said he would.

On Wednesday night Valerie talked to me about her husband. "Do you know what he says when you leave? He says, 'Don't die. Don't die.' "

I asked her, "Have you ever done anything for yourself in your life?"

"No."

"Then it's perfectly all right to die," I said. "But, before you die, I'd like you to straighten out your relationship with your husband."

I came back later that night. Valerie was out of bed. Pointing toward her husband, who was standing by the window, she said, "I just told him a few things, some of which he didn't want to hear."

On Thursday morning she was looking wonderful, and she said, "I have two questions. Where did all this energy come from? And why aré the nurses in my room all the time now?"

I told her, "The nurses are in your room because you're not dying anymore, and the energy comes from resolving your conflict with your husband. I don't know if a miracle will happen, but I think you should get up and go home."

"That is a little scary," she said. "I thought I was supposed to die today!"

Tests have shown a significant delay in nurses' responses to so-called terminal patients. However, this is not meant to be a derogatory statement about nurses. They must face their own mortality when they enter a room where somebody is labeled "dying," a difficulty we all face until we're comfortable with our own mortality.

Valerie's remission lasted for two or three months (a "little miracle"), during which she lived at home, accomplishing beautiful things with her family. She then died peacefully at home, surrounded by love. This example did more for the nursing staff than any number of lectures. They all saw what happens when someone resolves conflicts and finds new energy to heal. If we could do this with all our patients at an earlier stage, not only would they live longer and better, but we would probably increase the number of self-induced cures dramatically.

It's amazing how seldom members of the hospital staff visit patients who are close to death. If you shut the door, no one comes in.

I was once even questioned about killing someone because of this fear of seeing death. I was in a meeting when I received a call from Muriel, a young woman almost unable to breathe and near death from extensive cancer. She told me, "You say dying's easy. I looked up at the sky and said, 'I'm ready,' and nothing happened."

So I explained, "It's because you're too agitated. I can't get there till five o'clock, but then I'll come and help you." If patients want to wait they will.

When I came in, she was filled with fear and anger, and had been given no sedation. I tried to tell her that it is hard to die angry and fearful. It keeps you oriented to your body. You have to relax and let go. Then I asked for some morphine, enough to calm her and ease her pain.

Because of Muriel's youth, this was a frightening scene for the nurses. They had to be thinking, "This could be one of us in that bed." Only a brave medical student was there besides me and the patient's family. After the morphine took effect, her breathing became easier and we had a wonderful couple of hours, filled with love and laughter. She literally came alive again, and at one point said she'd be coming back as the first woman President.

By seven o'clock Muriel looked so much better that I

thought maybe she was changing her mind. I asked her, "Do you mind if I go get dinner?" She said no. I came back in half an hour, and she had died. I know that was her way of making it easier for me.

The nurses had announced she had died, but, when I walked into the room, Muriel's eyes were open, the intravenous pump was still running, and everything else was connected, as though she were still alive. The nurses had difficulty dealing with her death.

Later that night I heard that one of the nurses had called an administrator and said I might have killed a patient with morphine. The administrator wouldn't call me, because he wasn't an M.D. So it worked its way up to the medical chief of staff, who was at a party.

The next day the chief of staff, who knows me well, called me, and I explained what had happened. But the part that pained me was the nurse's inability to come into that room. She would have seen how beautiful Muriel's last hours were. These hours are gifts of love that help all the survivors go on. A patient of mine who died recently left me a note saying, "Thank you for the love. I *can* take it with me." She healed me and her family and all who touched her.

The love that flows from a life ended at peace was beautifully expressed in a poem by Juliet Burch, now a student at St. John's College. It was written at the bedside of her father, who died two days later.

> Sitting with Pa
> The man who was/is my father
> His laboured, rhythmical breathing
> The slightness of his stature now
> I hold his warm hand and
> The room is peaceful
> There is such a lack
> of fear
> in this room. It is a
> peaceful place to die.
> I am
> finally
> unafraid to hold the hand of a man who

was so mighty.
Meditation
A room that is
difficult to come to,
yet somehow
hard to leave.
His opened eye.
He is there
but what happens inside him?
A pause in the metronome of breath
I come to attention.
And then the rhythm
like the tired clock
returns.
I wonder if he is
crying
inside. Is he afraid
at all?
I worry less—
for I look to discover that
now the hand
being held
is mine.

The contrast between a natural, peaceful death and a
death artificially prolonged without dignity has been captured
in a similar poem by Joan Neet George.

Grandmother, When Your Child Died

Grandmother, when your child died
hot beside you
in your narrow bed,
his labored breathing kept
you restless
and woke you when
it sighed,
and stopped.

You held him through the bitter dawn
and in the morning

dressed him, combed his hair,
your tears welled, but you didn't weep
until at last he lay
among the wild iris in the sod,
his soul gone inexplicably to God. Amen.

But grandmother, when my child died
sweet Jesus, he died hard.
A motor beside
his sterile cot
groaned, and hissed, and whirred
while he sang his pain—
low notes and high notes
in slow measures
slipping through the drug-cloud.
My tears, redundant,
dropped slow
like glucose or blood
from a bottle.
And when he died
my eyes were dry
and gods wearing white coats
turned away.

NEW MEANING IN LIFE AND DEATH

There's a story about two businessmen who were driving
to an important meeting. Each was to receive $50,000 tax free,
but they had to get there in one hour. On the way, each had
a flat tire. The first businessman got out, looked in the trunk,
and found he had no jack. He looked at his watch, saw that he
had to reach his appointment within ten minutes, and had a
heart attack on the spot. The other businessman looked in the
trunk and also saw he had no jack. He stood by the car. A
passerby stopped, changed his tire for him, and he made his
appointment in time.

I subscribe to the Jungian idea of synchronicity, or meaningful coincidence. I believe that there are very few accidents.
After one of my talks a man handed me a card on which was

written, "Coincidence is God's way of remaining anonymous." In a life out of harmony with itself, events seem to conspire to go wrong, but by the same token they mesh wondrously when you start to live your bliss. Don't climb the ladder of success only to find that when you reach the top it is leaning against the wrong wall. As you begin living *your* life, taking risks to do what you really want to do, you will find things fall into place and you "just happen" to be in the right place at the right time. Even elevator doors start to open when you arrive.

Perhaps this is another way of saying you create your own opportunities out of the same raw materials from which other people create their defeats. I call these apparent setbacks "spiritual flat tires"—unexpected events that can have positive or negative outcomes, depending on how we respond to them. For example, a half-hour delay might save you from being in a traffic accident, or someone who stops to help you change a flat tire might turn out to be someone you needed to meet. Such occurrences teach us to stop judging events as necessarily good or bad, right or wrong, and instead just let life flow. A parent with cancer may be worrying about the effect on their child. If an author's best source is an unhappy childhood, perhaps a future best seller will come out of the pain, thus helping others and providing financial success. We can only decide what to do with our pain. That is our only option.

Let me give you another example of what I mean. One morning Rose, a student who worked with me, got into her car to come help me in the operating room. Her car broke down, so she got on her bike, and it broke. At that point she said to herself, "Well, according to Bernie, I belong back in my apartment." She went back, and as she entered her apartment, the phone rang.

It was her brother, a former drug addict, calling from Maine. He said, "Thank God you're there. I was just about to head for New York and go back on drugs." They talked for about an hour. She calmed him, and he promised to stay until another family member could go and be with him.

She then went out to her car and lifted the hood, saying to herself, "I don't know why I'm doing this. I don't know anything about engines." At that moment her other brother drove up and said, "I was driving down the parkway, and a voice said to me, 'Go by your sister's house.' " He fixed her car, and she came to the hospital with her eyes wide open. She will never need another sermon again.

To become an authentic, spiritual person means to open to our intuition, the part of us that *knows*. As Elisabeth Kübler-Ross has said, decisions based on cold reason alone are usually made to satisfy others. Intuitive decisions make *us* feel good, even if others think we're crazy. But, as we become authentic, we no longer worry about what others think.

A woman named Connie, a math teacher at our children's school, developed Hodgkin's disease. Her husband divorced her, and she was left with a mortgage and a teaching position, and was afraid to make any changes or moves. I talked to her, sent books to her, and tried to get her to redirect her life. One night at a PTA meeting I decided to get on line to talk to her, even though she was no longer our children's teacher. As I entered her room, she said, "I was looking for you." I said, "I know. That's why I'm here."

We sat down, and she said, "You know, I decided to do what you were telling me to do. One of the things that has interested me is taking flying lessons. So I started to. One Sunday at two o'clock I went out to the airport, and this handsome man stepped off another airplane. I thought, Boy! I could go for him, and to make a long story short, we're getting married, and I'm moving away with him."

I said, "What got you to the airport at two o'clock on Sunday? Why didn't you take a lesson at one o'clock on Saturday?" And we both laughed. It's doing what feels right to you that brings your life to fruition. It shows you all the people who are there to be loved and to love you, people whom you never saw before even though they were always there.

After hearing one of my talks, a man named Aaron came up to me and said he just couldn't believe his life had any spiritual guidance. He didn't have the faith that things would work out if he only had the courage to take the direction he really wanted. He was very unhappy with his house and his job. He wanted desperately to change both but was afraid to let go of the old and seek the new. I promised him, "If you just leave your job, another one will appear."

"Okay," he said, "I'll see," and he quit. Sunday he went to church, something he rarely did, and the man sitting next to him said, "I hear you left your job." Aaron said yes and told him the kind of work he did—and the man said, "I need someone just like you." Aaron was hired.

"Well," he told me, "you have to admit that could be a coincidence."

So I told him, "Now sell your house, and you'll find another one." He put the house on the market, but no one bought it. He had scheduled a tag sale to dispose of some of the furnishings, but he'd decided to cancel it because no one seemed interested in the house. However, I encouraged him to go ahead and hold the tag sale. One of the customers asked Aaron why he was holding the sale.

"I'm trying to sell this house, but I need another one," Aaron replied.

The customer told him, "Well, I'm selling a house that you might be interested in." It turned out to be exactly what Aaron was looking for. He bought it and soon sold his.

But again, you have to admit, this could be a coincidence. If one has no faith, then of course these are always coincidences. How do you know if you have faith? The only way I can explain it is to tell you about the man who fell over the side of a cliff, grabbed hold of a very small bush, and was hanging there, watching its roots gradually pull loose. At that moment he looked up toward heaven and said, "God, you have to save me." And a beautiful melodious voice said, "Don't worry, my son, I'll save you. Let go." The man looked back up and said, "Is anybody else up there?" If you don't have to ask that second question, you have faith.

As a healer I'm trying to get people to have faith in their own lives and in the whole process of life. You can act from that faith and make the rest of your life simple, or you can keep testing and make the rest of your life difficult. No matter what good things happen, you'll always be able to say, "It could be a coincidence," and never enjoy the grace. Instead I counsel you to choose your direction, make the leap of faith, and fly.

Let the occasional spiritual flat tires redirect your life. That's what survivors do. They don't have failures. They have delays or redirections.

Choosing spiritual guidance also helps you to see that people's minds and souls are interconnected in ways normally obscured from our everyday vision. The separateness most of us experience is illusory, and seeing through it makes life even more meaningful. Botanist Rupert Sheldrake has recently proposed "morphogenetic fields" as a means of communication to explain the otherwise baffling results of certain experiments. It seems that, once rats in one laboratory have learned a particular maze, other rats *anywhere in the world*, having had no contact with the original rats, learn that same maze faster. Apparently, once a thought has been thought, it can be communicated to others. Sheldrake believes this may be the reason why an important discovery is often made simultaneously by several people working independently in different areas of the world.

There are hidden channels of communication from the unconscious to our conscious minds. As I previously mentioned, Jung has written, "The future is unconsciously prepared long in advance, and therefore can be guessed by clairvoyants." Since I've made patients understand that it's safe to tell me *any* experience they've had, I've encountered cases of precognition many times. Some patients draw or describe the exact details of upcoming surgery, down to the precise placement of equipment and personnel, despite having no knowledge of the room or the procedure.

Several years ago I was asked to see Janet, a pregnant woman whose husband had just been killed in an auto accident. At one point during our conversation, I said, "Your husband knew he was going to die."

"Do you really believe that?" she asked.

"I certainly do."

It gave her some comfort, for then she understood better why her husband had insisted she become independent by earning a nursing degree. She also recalled that, several weeks before her husband's death, they'd been talking about accidents, and he said, "If I ever have brain damage, I wouldn't want to live. I can lose an arm or a leg and I would still go on, but if I have brain damage I wouldn't want to live." The autopsy had shown extensive brain damage.

I also told Janet I believed her husband's spirit exists. Again she asked, "Do you really believe that?" And I said, "Yes, I do."

"Well," she said, "I was sitting in the living room. He was late for dinner, and the town fire alarm went off. I knew it was about him. I jumped up, and his voice came to me and said, 'Do not leave the room for one hour.' So I sat down and waited. When I got to the scene of the accident, they were just lifting his body out of the car. I thought to myself, 'If I had been out here for an hour, I would never have survived.'"

I worried about her but several months later I mentioned her story in a conference on drawings, and a physician who was there told me he'd delivered her child and she had done beautifully. Recently Janet wrote me a letter, offering her help to anyone in a crisis similar to what she had survived.

This physician also beckoned me over to a corner and told me of a precognitive experience. While his wife was pregnant she had said to him, "I must study total communication for the deaf." He said, "Honey, why do you need to do that?" She said, "I must." And of course their first child was born deaf. So the physician was a believer, but he had motioned for me to come into a corner to talk about this. I know that finger waggle from many physicians. It means, "I agree with you, but I'm uncomfortable revealing it in front of others."

Time after time in my experiences with patients I encounter unconscious knowledge of the future. One Monday I operated on a man named Mike, who had a massive hemorrhage from an aneurysm that had ruptured into his esophagus. It was impossible to stop the bleeding, and he died. When I talked to his wife, she said, "You know, Sunday we spent the whole day discussing his funeral and will, and I said, 'Why do we have to talk about all this morbid business?' And now I know."

Several times I've found that close relatives knew of a person's death before they had received news of it. My own father, who is now almost eighty, told me a few years ago that his mother visited him—spiritually—one day at work when he was a young man. She said good-bye. He knew she had died, and he grew terribly sad. His co-workers noticed, but he couldn't tell them what had .happened because it sounded crazy. As soon as he got home, the phone rang, and his sister told him their mother had died.

Sandy, whom I mentioned in Chapter 4, told me her experience of the same intuitive knowledge. Her husband, Harry, always drove the kids to school, but one day all three of them were late getting dressed. He got angry and left without them, and a few minutes later was killed in an accident. It seems obvious to me that there was an unconscious awareness in each of those children that this was not the day to get dressed and go with dad.

When Sandy called Harry's mother in Maine and started to talk, his mother said, "Yes, I know. Harry's dead." When asked how she knew, she replied, "His father"—who'd been dead a year—"came to me last night and said, 'I have to take our son tomorrow.'" These are the kinds of things that patients share with me, the privileged listener. They are experiences that can open a whole new realm in one's awareness and belief system.

One night, when I was giving a lecture, I had all my notes in front of me. And yet, as I was giving the talk, I realized that, in a sense, two talks were being given. In one, I was struggling to follow the outline, but something else was coming out of my mouth. I realized the other talk was much better, so I finally just gave in and let it happen.

When I came off the stage, I told Bobbie, "I don't know who gave that talk. I didn't." The next woman who came up to me said, "I've heard you before, but that was more moving than usual." The third person who came up to me said, "I'm a medium, and while you were reading Lois Becker's letter, superimposed over you and staring at the audience was this figure. I drew him for you." And she showed me a picture of my guide George.

The famous psychic Olga Worrell has also described George and another of my meditative guides, even including the clothes they wear—flowing robes and the old Jewish prayer caps. When the emotional and spiritual mind is freed, the distinctions between the "mystical" and the "mundane" break down.

This experience taught me that the unconscious can take care of everything, and I don't have to prepare for my lectures anymore. Whether George exists as a spiritual guide or simply exists inside of me as part of my collective unconscious or intuition, the power is there for all of us, if we will let it come through. As Socrates replied when asked if he had prepared his defense, "What needs to be said will be said."

One woman who had breast cancer told me that her family thought she was crazy. I asked why, and she told me several stories. One was a dream in which Death came and told her that her husband was going to die tomorrow. She argued with Death and said, "No. Everybody gets two weeks' notice." Two weeks to the day later her husband died.

I told her I loved her and all that she was sharing with me. When we went out of the examining room, her family was expecting me to say something negative about their crazy mother. Instead I said, "She's wonderful, terrific." That led to a new openness and awareness on the part of the family, a new willingness to accept her and all that she had shared with them.

Death is no barrier to this intuitive, spiritual consciousness. It continues after death, and it communicates between the dead and the living. Iris, a blind diabetic who developed cancer, underwent a similar experience. One day she called her two daughters into her hospital room and told them, "Girls, I can see again. My mother and father came for me and held out an apple. They said when I bite into it I will join them. I told them my grandson's birthday was on Tuesday, and I would join them then." She died after the party on Tuesday.

Before she passed away, one of her daughters said, "Mom, if you die I want to die, too. I can't go on without you." Two weeks later Iris appeared to her daughter and said, "Look, I have ten minutes. This is against the rules. I am in a beautiful place and I am loved. I can't be worrying about you doing something silly."

As I have opened myself to my patients' beliefs, I have received many messages from those who have died. Josie was a wonderful woman who had given everyone who knew her the gift of love and humor. While at the hospice, for example, she thought she heard a noise and asked if someone was at the door. The nurse said, "Oh, I just kicked your bucket." Josie replied, "I'm here *trying* to kick the bucket, and for you it's easy." She was one of the exceptional people who lived until the moment of death.

Josie had asked me to deliver the eulogy at her funeral. I said I would be honored, but told her I couldn't be sure my schedule would permit it, especially since the funeral would be held in New York. Months before, I had arranged to be in New York on a certain Friday for a conference. The only day in the entire year I was scheduled to be in New York. Then a radio talk show host asked me to speak for an hour at noon on that day, since I would already be in the city. I agreed, but on the Monday before the show someone from the station called and said the program had been preempted. I told my wife that Josie's funeral would be at that time although she hadn't died yet.

On Tuesday evening, Josie's husband asked me how to help ease her passage. She found it hard to leave amid the constant visiting and expressions of love. I suggested he tell her he loved her, that he and the boys would be okay, and she could go if she was ready. He shared that with her the next morning, and then turned to get her breakfast tray. When he turned back, she had died.

Josie's son called me to tell me she had died, and that there had been a debate about whether to have the funeral Friday or Sunday. I said, "Your mother wants it at noon on Friday." He said, "I don't know how you know, but that's what we decided."

After I'd learned of Josie's death, I went to meditate in the hospital chapel, a small closet-like room with no windows. A plaque on the wall suddenly began to shake for no discernible reason. I looked at it and read the message: "In the midst of life I am with you." I knew it was a message from Josie. On Friday, as I was nearing the end of my eulogy, the loudspeaker in the funeral home suddenly went off. I felt that was another message from Josie, saying, "Enough already!"

Paula, one of our ECaP group members, told me of a similar experience after her daughter was murdered in a brutal assault at her college. At the murderer's trial, a bird appeared in the window, making an awful racket and disturbing the proceedings. Paula said she knew it was her daughter, because she always demanded a lot of attention. Later at the wedding of Paula's other daughter, another bird appeared, cackling raucously, interrupting the outdoor ceremony. Then, after Paula finished telling this story in the group, a bird began squawking at the window, and everyone turned to Paula and said, "I guess that's your daughter again."

Recently I was out jogging on a cold, dark December morning. A bird followed me for half an hour, chirping and sharing with me. When I came home, I said to Bobbie, "Someone died and just said good-bye." Wednesday I got a phone call and learned that a patient I'd been very close to, who was in another state, had died at that time.

Perhaps my most dramatic experience of after-death communication concerns Bill, the physician I mentioned in Chapter 2, who knew he had cancer after one instance of difficulty in swallowing. He joined ECaP but always remained somewhat distant—quiet and observant. His wife had told others, "He never bought the package."

Three months after Bill had died of his cancer, a young college student came to my office to interview me. She said she'd been in a healing circle the night before, and since they knew she was going to see me the next day, the medium who was directing the circle had asked if there was any message for me. She handed me a card:

> To Bernie
> From Bill
> With love and peace
> If I had known it was
> this easy, I'd have bought
> the package a long time ago
> and wouldn't have
> resisted so much.

When I called his wife, she said, "That's what he always told me after the meetings. He would attend, but he said he couldn't buy the package." When he was quite sick, I asked him if he was ready to die. He said, "Considering the alternative, no." The people in the healing circle knew nothing about who Bill was, yet there was the same phrase he and his wife used. "Love and peace" is the closing I use for all my letters. Who else could this note be from? How can I help but believe and share this belief with others? As Elisabeth Kübler-Ross says, "One day all my critics will agree with me."

But, whatever explanation you prefer for these experiences, there's no denying that learning to love conquers the fear of death, and can liberate incredible healing energy. The closing lines of Emmet Foxes' sermon are the key. "If only you could love enough, you would be the happiest and most powerful being in the world . . ." You become invulnerable. This, I feel, is the real future of medicine. Scientists often say you must see in order to believe, but I know you must believe in order to see. When I was in college and took philosophy and religion, one day the teacher was discussing St. Augustine, who said you must love in order to see. I raised my hand and said, "I thought love was blind." I never got a satisfactory answer from the teacher. Now I see that you must love and believe, that is, be open, so that true sharing can occur, and you will see what is in front of you. In medicine and science, we are generally told, "Seeing is believing," and then we are told what to see, and to ignore everything else. However, the spiritual message heeded by the true explorer or artist is to open our eyes and see beyond what we have been told exists.

It is my fervent hope that, by showing adults how the mind and spirit can heal the body and make life worthwhile, I can help us, as parents, raise a generation of children programmed to be loving and healthy. Too many children get everything they want and nothing they need. The message to whisper in your child's ear is simply, "I love you unconditionally (not *if* you get an A, or become a doctor). Life is full of hurdles, but whatever happens, you'll overcome." Then give them some discipline, not punishment. In Soviet Georgia, people drink a toast "To your three-hundredth birthday." We should adopt the same custom.

The whole world must confront the same issues, for nuclear weapons threaten the world as cancer threatens the individual. If we decide to love, we have a much greater chance of surviving. If we love, we will control the few who are comfortable being killers. As Gandhi said, "We must not kill our enemies, but kill their desire to kill."

In India the story is told of a holy man who stayed in his monastery when an army was advancing through the area and killing all the holy men. When a general said, "Don't you know I can thrust my sword into your stomach?" he replied, "Don't you know I can place my stomach around your sword?" If we love enough, we become invulnerable, and we can place our stomachs around the sword and save the world. In India there is also this traditional saying: "When you were born, you cried and the world rejoiced. Live your life in such a manner that when you die the world cries and you rejoice." If we can live in accordance with that simple teaching, we will survive as individuals, and the world will survive as well. As George Ritchie wrote at the conclusion of his book *Return from Tomorrow*, "God is busy building a race of men who know how to love. I believe that the fate of the earth itself depends on the progress we make—and that the time now is very short."

Gandhi's teacher Muktananda remarked that Sanskrit has no word for *exclusion*. When we can kill our own desire to kill, and learn to exclude no one, the world will change, and we will return from whence we came—from the energy that chose to love out of its own intelligence.

I often tell my patients there are two ways to be immortal. One is to go to medical school (Doctors don't get sick and don't die). And the other is to love someone.

As Thornton Wilder expressed it at the end of *The Bridge of San Luis Rey:*

And we ourselves shall be loved for a while and forgotten. But the love will have been enough; all those impulses of love return to the love that made them. Even memory is not necessary for love. There is a land of the living and a land of the dead, and the bridge is love, the only survival, the only meaning.

God has given us free will to make love and life meaningful. This creates a critical risk because we now have the ability to destroy our universe if we choose not to love.

However, it is only in this critical time that the archetype of the miracle can appear. When one believes in love and miracles divine intervention can occur.

We have an infinite number of choices ahead, but a finite number of endings. They are destruction and death or love and healing. If we choose the path of love we save ourselves and our universe.

Let us choose love and life.

Appendix

RELAXATION

The following method, given in the Simontons' book *Getting Well Again*, was adapted by Dr. Edmond Jacobson from a yoga technique. Instructions can also be found in Larry LeShan's *How to Meditate* and Herbert Benson's *The Relaxation Response*. As with the examples of imaging later on, you are encouraged to have a friend speak these instructions to you, or record them yourself on tape. A tape is always available to you in times of stress. The tape is also useful if you fall asleep, because you are still hearing the message. I don't recommend that you use it to fall asleep, however, unless you need help to relax at night. During the day, just take any comfortable position and try to listen to it in its entirety. With practice, you may often be able to enter the alpha state by yourself without the tape.

Adjust the lighting so it is soft and restful. If possible, at least in the beginning, use a quiet room and close the door so you will not be interrupted. This alone says you are important, that you are willing to take the time for healing. However, a quiet room is not always essential. Familiar noises may actually be restful, indicating you are in a safe environment. Using the same place each time is helpful. Just getting into a favorite chair can immediately set the mood and lead to rapid relaxation. You may find it helpful to play some gentle, soothing music—at low volume. There are also many prerecorded meditation tapes and records available that can help you. I especially recommend Pachelbel's *Canon* in the recording by Daniel Kobialka. Be sure these instructions from the Simonton book are spoken quietly and slowly, with pauses where appropriate.

Take a comfortable position in a chair, with your feet flat on the floor, or lying down on a couch or mat. Feel the pleasant pressure of the chair or other surface on your buttocks and back.

Gently pay attention to your breathing as you let your breaths come in a natural rhythm, without hurrying them or trying to slow them.

Now take a few calm, deep breaths, and as you exhale, think the words "relax, let go."

Direct your attention to your face, eyes, and jaw. Feel whatever tension is concentrated there. Now make a mental image of that tension, such as a coiled spring, a stretched rubber band, a block of ice melting, or a rope tied in a knot. Then picture that tense object relaxing, uncoiling, loosening. Feel that relaxation in every part of your face. Momentarily contract every muscle in your face, squeeze your eyes and mouth tightly shut, then let them relax as you continue to see your spring, rubber band, or rope becoming limp.

Experience the relaxation in your face as the beginning of a wave that is spreading throughout your body. You may experience this wave as a sensation of heaviness, lightness, or tingling, of pleasant warmth or (in the summer) delicious coolness. Move your mind now to each area of your body—your neck, shoulders, arms, hands and fingers, chest, back, abdomen, hips and genitals, thighs, lower legs, all the way down to your feet and toes. Momentarily tense each part, then let go as you concentrate on your mental image of relaxation. Experience the wave of relaxation spreading throughout your body as you do this. Then remain in this peaceful state for five minutes or so.

When you are ready to arise, simply let your mind focus on the sounds in the room, gradually let your eyelids become lighter, then open your eyes. Slowly get up and notice how you can combine the feeling of relaxation with the alertness needed for your everyday activities.

If your mind wanders or you feel tense, you have two choices. You can respond to the thoughts that are leading your mind astray, such as "Did I leave the dishwasher on?" You can go look, then come back and finish your meditation. Or you can decide not to answer those thoughts, and let go of them. Just remember that relaxation will quickly become easier with practice, then guide your mind gently back to the spoken directions.

GUIDED VISUALIZATIONS

You yourself, a friend, a family member, or a therapist can lead you in visualization. Here are some sample visualizations that can easily be adapted to your particular needs. Simply have someone you love and trust speak the words in a calm, gentle voice, or speak them yourself into a tape recorder, then play the tape as you meditate. Speak slowly and carefully, and be sure to make the pauses long enough to fully experience the images visualized. The pauses I've marked should be at least 15 to 20 seconds. Where I suggest a long pause, allow at least 30 to 60 seconds. The pauses can be longer, and you need not follow the voice continuously. You may need to follow other imagery that appears in your consciousness. You may include:

1. going to a masquerade.
2. participating in a circus.
3. moving through a dark tunnel and emerging into the light to be greeted by family and significant others.
4. experiencing holding on and letting go physically and emotionally.
5. seeing yourself as a child when sad and happy, and how you as an adult respond to that child.
6. achieving your chosen career, and what it means to you.
7. confronting fears or choices present in your life and seeing a successful outcome.
8. performing for others on stage and seeing their reaction.
9. floating in healing water.
10. rowing with others helping you and building your support system.
11. finding a message or gift in the depths of a pond.
12. being reborn.
13. weaving the fabric of your life.

The choices are limitless and your own unconscious is your best therapist.

I refer those who are interested in pursuing hypnotic techniques further to the work of Dr. Milton Erickson.

Each session can be introduced and/or accompanied by music or sounds of nature, such as a recording of the ocean, that you find especially relaxing. Just be sure to keep the volume low enough during the meditation itself so as not to distract you from the spoken words or the images in your mind. You may want to use one of our ECaP tapes, recorded with background music. If you or a friend plan to record your own tape, I suggest you use two tape recorders. Play some soft, soothing music, such as Pachelbel's *Canon*, on one machine, while recording both the music and the voice on the other.

The visualization sessions do take time, but this is a "live" message. You are worth the time. Thus I recommend that most of my patients do them three or more times a day and take fifteen minutes at three or more other times throughout the day for quieting relaxation. The benefits spill over into the hours afterward, and you maintain a reserve of calm while facing the stress of other activities. The ideal is going through the whole day in a sort of guided trance, so that serenity remains at all times. We should try to be like Danielle, a patient who told me, "I meditate all day. If I wash the dishes, I think of my cancer being washed out of my body. If I take a walk and a breeze blows, I see it blown away." She connects everything she does back to healing.

A hypnotherapist can be valuable in the beginning, especially if the patient has trouble entering the state of deep relaxation. No matter who sets the course for the first meditative sessions—doctor, counselor, hypnotherapist, or the patient—care should be taken to appeal to the person's dominant sense. In other words, for someone who responds to the world primarily through the eyes, the guided imagery should consist mainly of visual images—seeing a rose in all its color and beauty. If the person is auditory-dominant, as most musicians are, the directions should appeal to the ear—hearing a bee buzzing in the center of the rose. Those who place great emphasis on the olfactory sense should concentrate on smelling the rose. For those with a tactile, "hands-on" approach to the world, touch and feeling need to be emphasized—the rose's silken petals.

Remember that you do not have to follow the voice. If you are experiencing some significant imagery of your own, stay with it while the voice goes on. You'll be able to catch up with the voice later.

A problem often arises when patients try to visualize their disease as receding when laboratory tests tell them it's spreading. They may be unable to keep the image clear, or they may feel as though they're lying to themselves. It's crucial to remember the difference between an objective picture and the desired outcome, between the present and the future. The images represent *what you want to happen*, and there is no contradiction between seeing your hopes clearly and facing the facts of the present. The more clearly you can see the future you desire, the more likely it is to come true.

Visualization 1

Take a comfortable position. It's generally better to uncross hands and feet, so there's no pressure. Begin to become aware of your breathing, and the motion of your chest and abdomen as you breathe deeply in and out. Sometimes repeating a word like "peace" or "relax" to yourself with each breath will help. Just deep breaths, letting the peace in and the tension out. And the music, and my voice, and the sounds in the room will all help relax you. When you're ready, you may look upward and let your eyes close gently, although you may do this meditation with your eyes open, if you like. Unwind, erase the blackboard of your mind, and just feel yourself settling down. Perhaps let a wave of peace move down through your body, relaxing the tense muscles, particularly the neck and shoulder muscles, and the jaw muscles, then moving down your body, through your chest and abdomen, and gradually into your lower extremities. Your body may feel heavy or warm, or it may tingle. It may help to give the wave a color, and let it move down. [Pause]

And then into your mind's eye allow a pleasant scene to appear. This is going to be your special little corner of the universe off in the middle of nowhere. I'd like you to create all the vivid colors that you know are there, as well as the textures, the aromas, and the sounds that you will associate with it. And how you feel here is perfectly all right, for it's a safe place for you. It's yours. Take a moment to find a spot where you can sit or lie down. And if there is any illness within your body, see your treatment and your immune system eliminating that illness from your body. If there is no illness present, just see your body rejecting illness. See yourself becoming well and becoming the person you'd like to be. Take a moment to help make yourself well. [Long pause]

When you have completed the healing process, I want you to follow my voice again, and build a bridge from your corner of the universe to mine. It'll connect with a path. Look at that bridge you've built, and see what it's like. And then come across to the path. It's covered with smooth gravel, and you'll feel that under your feet. There's warm sunlight, broken up by the shade of trees. And just come down the path with me. If the path divides, just take the right turn. Continue to take the right turn whenever the path divides.

Ahead of you, you will see five steps. With each step down you'll feel more relaxed and more at peace. Then ahead of you on the right will be a lovely garden. Enter the garden. Enjoy the aromas, and perhaps touch a petal. See the beauty that exists. Perhaps even hear the birds or other animals that may be living there. I'd like you to pick out one flower and observe its individuality and beauty, and see how much it resembles you in your individuality and beauty. [Pause]

Then I'd like you to picture yourself as a seed. And I'm going to plant you in nice warm earth about an inch below the surface. You'll feel the moisture and the sun warming you. I want you to grow and bloom. Break out of that seed and observe yourself breaking forth, and growing, and blooming. Watch the process happen. [Long pause]

When you have bloomed and become that beautiful flower, find a place inside you to store it. Make it a part of you.

Then I'd like you to follow me along the path again. Ahead of you, you'll see an enormous rainbow-colored balloon, with a gondola or basket hanging from it. I want you to climb into the basket and release the balloon. There's nothing to fear, it's very safe. It'll float upwards through the clouds, past the birds, all sounds relaxing you, all sounds bringing peace. [Pause]

And as you move higher, you will eventually achieve an astronaut's view of the earth. What a feeling of peace that brings! What can make it even more peaceful is to find the pad and pencil that are in the basket, and write down on the pad those conflicts or problems that exist in your life. [Pause]

Then take that paper, crumple it, and leave it in orbit. Cast it behind you. Feel the difference in how light you feel and how easily you float on with those problems left behind. Take a moment now to just float onward, totally at peace, totally free of concerns, weightless. [Long pause]

Then, when you've completed that, you may follow my voice again, and come back down, further down, descending, slowly, back to the place we started. Be careful climbing out, because you're very relaxed. I'd like you to lie there now, in a meadow next to the path. And just take a moment to fill your body with love. Open every cell and fill it with love. [Pause]

Now step out of yourself for a minute, and look back at yourself. Give yourself the love and affection you deserve. And then step back into your body. And listen to it. Go through your body and listen. Listen to each organ. What is it telling you? What music does it make? Are you in harmony? For those parts that aren't, give them a little extra love. Open every cell to love. See if you can create a healing harmony within yourself. If there are any areas of pain, any areas you usually don't pay attention to, I would give them an extra measure of love. [Long pause]

Now just let your awareness of your body begin to increase, perhaps noting the position you're in, the pressure the chair or floor makes against your body, the motion of your chest and abdomen as you breathe deeply in and out. And let this awareness begin to increase as you get closer to coming back to the room. Perhaps wiggling your fingers and toes will help. [Pause]

Then, count seven to ten breaths after my voice stops, each breath making you feel lighter, more awake, more alert, yet still at peace, until after the last breath you open your eyes and return to the room when you're ready, beginning now.

Visualization 2

Take a comfortable position. And let the conflict flow out, and just unwind, relax, and think peace. As you breathe deeply, let peace come in. Perhaps visualize a beautiful rainbow, and relax with each breath. Once again settle down, and let that wave of color move down through your body, bringing peace. Let your eyes close if you want to. Take a moment to just fill your body with love and peace. Don't overlook any places, particularly those parts and organs that may be involved with disease. [Long pause]

When you're done, take yourself to your corner of the universe, that lovely, vivid place with its aromas and textures, familiar sounds and colors. And just be there, taking a moment to allow the warmth of the sun and the energy of the earth to heal you, to be safe and at peace here. Just settle down, down. You might picture yourself being on an elevator, descending floor by floor, feeling more relaxed with each floor. [Long pause]

Then I'd like you to build that bridge again, to my part of the universe, where all the people you know and deal with live. And I'd like you to invite them across that bridge, those you love and those you have conflict with, those you don't like. Bring them all together in your little corner of the universe. And bring them *together,* to touch, to hug, to share, and say, "I love you." And watch the transformation. [Long pause]

Then you may leave them, and follow my voice. I'm going to bring you across the bridge again, along the path. Once again you may experience the familiar crunch of the gravel, the path, the sunlight, the meadows. [Pause]

Once again you come to the steps down, feeling more relaxed with each step. [Pause]

You'll notice in front of you a great big sign, with paint cans and brushes around. The sign is empty. On the other side of the path is a big stone with a chisel and hammer. And I'd like you to leave a message for those who come after you, either by painting or by carving. Take a moment now to leave a message. [Long pause]

Then, when you're done, come down the path again. Ahead of you, you'll see an enormous old house, which I'd like you to enter. There'll be a lovely recliner sitting in the living room, and I'd like you to lie down on it. See yourself resting there and relaxing. You're becoming deeply relaxed and very much at peace. [Pause]

In that relaxed state I'd like you to walk through the house, because in one of the rooms there will be a chest, and within it is a meaningful message or gift for you. So explore the house, and find that message or gift. Find the message that lies within your chest. [Long pause]

When you're done, I'd like you to go back to the living room and lie down on that recliner again. I'd like you to take a moment to explore all the rooms and hallways of your mind and brain. You'll find one room that has to do with the immune system, another having to do with circulation, another with emotion, and so on. [Pause]

If you're dealing with disease, I'd like you to go into the rooms having to do with the immune system and circulation, and turn the right valves, and push the right switches, so that any disease in your body is healed, and the nourishment for that disease is turned off. Take a moment now to utilize those controls and help your body get well. [Long pause]

Once that's completed—you may stay if you're still working on it—come back out on the path again. As you walk out along the path, I'd like you to see, way off in the distance, a very bright white-yellow light. Coming out of that light, you'll see someone. As this person gets closer, you'll begin to see his or her appearance. Finally, this person will be close enough for you to ask his or her name, and know that this person is a guide for you, someone you can always call on to help you. [Pause]

Sit down for a moment with your guide along the path, and question your guide about some conflict or problem, and see what advice you get. [Long pause]

When you have completed that conference, I'd like you to follow me again—but if you haven't completed it, stay and talk. Know that you can always call upon your guide at any time. If you are done, you may follow me over a hill. On the other side you will see a beach. There are several gulls floating by, beautiful ocean waves, the warm sand. I want to teach you how to fly, just as the gulls do. But first I want you to think of your problems and give them a weight, and put them on your back. And then take three steps forward, and with the third step rise up and fly. One . . . two . . . three and up. Feel what it's like to fly with that weight. Then turn and let the weight fall off. And feel the difference when you let go of your problems. And just enjoy flying now. Let the sun warm you, and let the breeze hold you up and heal you. There's no effort. From now on, at any time of stress you can recall flying and feeling free, casting your problems away, dropping them off your shoulders. Just round off your shoulders and let them slide. [Long pause]

And then allow yourself to come down on the sand again. Stretch out, and allow the energy of the earth and the warmth of the sunlight to heal you. Once again take a moment to open your body to love. Open each cell, each organ. Create your own music, your own harmony, your own beauty. Give all parts of yourself the love and affection they deserve. [Long pause]

When you have completed that, just let your body awareness begin to return—the chair, your position, your feet on the floor, all of these feelings. Gradually move parts of your body to awaken them, coming back feeling awake and alert and comfortable. Again use your breathing to bring you back up, counting seven breaths, feeling one seventh more awake and more alert with each breath, until you open your eyes and return to the room, starting now.

To order audio tapes of lectures by Dr. Siegel and meditation tapes, see pages 243–244.

READING LIST

Achterberg, Jeanne, and G. Frank Lawlis. *Imagery of Disease.* Institute for Personality and Ability Testing, Champaign, Ill 61820, 1978.

Ader, Robert, ed. *Psychoneuroimmunology.* Academic Press, New York, 1981.

Alexander, Franz. *Psychosomatic Medicine.* Norton, New York, 1965.

Bennett, Hal, and Mike Samuels. *The Well Body Book.* Random House, New York, 1973.

Benson, Herbert. *The Mind-Body Effect.* Simon & Schuster, New York, 1979; Berkley, New York, 1980.

Bresler, David E. and Richard Trubo. *Free Yourself from Pain.* Simon & Schuster, New York, 1979.

Breznitz, Shlomo, ed. *The Denial of Stress.* International Universities Press, New York, 1984.

Bry, Adelaide and Marjorie Blair. *Directing the Movies of Your Mind.* Harper & Row, New York, 1978.

Buscaglia, Leo. *Love.* Charles B. Slack, 6900 Grove Road, Thorofare, N.J. 08086, 1972; Fawcett Crest/Ballantine, New York, 1982.

———. *Living, Loving & Learning.* Charles B. Slack, 1982.

Capra, Fritjof. *The Tao of Physics.* Shambhala, Boulder, 1975; Bantam, New York, 1977.

Cousins, Norman. *Anatomy of an Illness as Perceived by the Patient.* Norton, New York, 1979; Bantam, New York, 1981.

Dowling, Colette. *The Cinderella Complex: Women's Hidden Fear of Independence.* Summit Books, New York, 1981; Pocket Books, New York, 1981.

Evans, Elida. *A Psychological Study of Cancer.* Dodd, Mead, New York, 1926.

Faraday, Ann. *Dream Power.* Berkley, New York, 1973.

Fosshage, James L., and Paul Olsen. *Healing: Implications for Psychotherapy.* Human Sciences Press, New York, 1978.

Fox, Emmet. *The Sermon on the Mount.* Harper & Row, New York, 1938.

Frankl, Viktor. *Man's Search for Meaning.* Pocket Books, New York, 1959, 1980.

Garfield, Charles, ed. *Psychosocial Care of the Dying Patient.* McGraw-Hill, New York, 1978.

Garfield, Patricia. *Creative Dreaming.* Simon & Schuster, New York, 1974; Ballantine, New York, 1976.

Glassman, Judith. *The Cancer Survivors: And How They Did It.* Doubleday, New York, 1983.

Green, Elmer, and Alyce Green. *Beyond Biofeedback.* Delacorte Press, New York, 1977.

Harris, Thomas A. *I'm OK—You're OK: A Practical Guide to Transactional Analysis.* Harper & Row, New York, 1969; Avon Books, New York, 1982.

Hutschnecker, Arnold. *The Will to Live.* Cornerstone Library, New York, 1951.

James, Muriel, and Dorothy Jongeward. *Born to Win.* Addison-Wesley, 1971; New American Library, New York, 1978.

Jampolsky, Gerald. *Love Is Letting Go of Fear.* Celestial Arts, 231 Adrian Road, Millbrae, Ca. 94030, 1979.

———, *Teach Only Love: The Seven Principles of Attitudinal Healing.* Bantam, New York, 1983.

————. *There Is a Rainbow Behind Every Dark Cloud.* Celestial Arts, Berkeley, CA, 1978.

Johnson, Robert A. *He: Understanding Masculine Psychology.* Harper & Row, New York, 1977.

————. *She: Understanding Feminine Psychology.* Harper & Row, New York, 1977.

Jung, Carl G. *Man and His Symbols.* Dell, New York, 1968.

————. *Memories, Dreams, Reflections.* Pantheon, New York, 1963; Vintage, New York, 1965.

————. *Modern Man in Search of a Soul.* Harcourt Brace Jovanovich, New York, 1955.

Kaufman, Barry N. *To Love Is to Be Happy With.* Fawcett, Greenwich, Conn., 1978.

Keleman, Stanley. *Living Your Dying.* Random House, New York, 1976.

Koller, Alice. *An Unknown Woman: A Journey to Self-Discovery.* Holt, Rinehart & Winston, New York, 1982.

Kruger, Helen. *Other Healers, Other Cures.* Bobbs-Merrill, Indianapolis, 1974.

Kübler-Ross, Elisabeth. *On Death and Dying.* Macmillan, New York, 1969.

————. *Death: The Final Stage of Growth.* Prentice-Hall, Englewood Cliffs, N.J., 1975.

————. *To Live Until We Say Goodbye.* Prentice-Hall, Englewood Cliffs, N.J., 1978.

Kushner, Harold S. *When Bad Things Happen to Good People.* Schocken, New York, 1981; Avon, New York, 1983.

Lair, Jess. *I Ain't Much, Baby, But I'm All I've Got.* Fawcett, Greenwich, Conn., 1978.

Landorf, Joyce. *Irregular People.* Word Books, Waco, TX, 1982.

Lappé, Frances Moore. *Diet for a Small Planet.* Random House, New York, 1971; Ballantine, New York, 1975.

Leonard, Jonathan N., J. L. Hofer, and Nathan Pritikin. *Live Longer Now: The First One Hundred Years of Your Life.* Grosset & Dunlap, New York, 1974.

LeShan, Lawrence L. *You Can Fight for Your Life: Emotional Factors in the Causation of Cancer.* Evans, New York, 1977.

————. *How to Meditate.* Little, Brown, Boston, 1974; Bantam, New York, 1975.

Lewis, Howard, and Martha E. Lewis. *Psychosomatics: How Your Emotions Can Damage Your Health.* Viking, New York, 1972.

Lingerman, Hal. *The Healing Energies of Music.* Theosophical Publishing House, Wheaton, Ill., 1983.

Locke, Steven, and Mady Hornig-Rohan. *Mind and Immunity.* Institute for the Advancement of Health, New York, 1983.

Matarazzo, J. D., et al. (eds.). *Behavioral Health.* John Wiley, New York, 1984.

Monroe, Robert. *Journeys Out of the Body.* Anchor/Doubleday, Garden City, N.Y., 1971.

Moody, Raymond A., Jr. *Life After Life.* Mockingbird Books, Box 110, Covington, Ga. 30209, 1975; Bantam, New York, 1976.

Müller, Robert. *Most of All, They Taught Me Happiness.* Doubleday, New York, 1978.

Nouwen, Henri. *Out of Solitude.* Ave Maria Press, Notre Dame, Ind., 1974.

———. *The Wounded Healer: Ministry in Contemporary Society.* Doubleday, New York, 1979.

———. *Genesee Diary: Report from a Trappist Monastery.* Doubleday, New York, 1981.

Ornstein, Robert E. *The Psychology of Consciousness.* First edition, W. H. Freeman, San Francisco, 1972; second edition, Harcourt Brace Jovanovich, New York, 1977.

Oyle, Irving. *The Healing Mind.* Pocket Books, New York, 1975.

———. *Time, Space & the Mind.* Celestial Arts, Berkeley, 1976.

Pelletier, Kenneth R. *Mind as Healer, Mind as Slayer.* Delacorte, New York, 1977; Delta, 1978.

———. *Toward a Science of Consciousness.* Delacorte Press, New York, 1978.

Progoff, Ira. *The Well and the Cathedral,* 2nd ed. Dialogue House Library, 80 E. 11th St., New York, N.Y. 10003, 1981.

———. *At a Journal Workshop: The Basic Text and Guide for Using the Intensive Journal.* Dialogue House Library, 80 E. 11th St., New York, N.Y. 10003, 1981.

Ritchie, George G., and Elizabeth Sherrill. *Return from Tomorrow.* Fleming H. Revell, 184 Central Ave., Old Tappan, N.J. 07675, 1981.

Rush, Anne K. *Getting Clear.* Random House, New York, 1973.

Samuels, Mike, and Nancy Samuels. *Seeing with the Mind's Eye.* Random House, New York, 1975.

Satir, Virginia M. *Peoplemaking.* Science & Behavior Books, P.O. Box 60519, Palo Alto, Ca. 94306, 1972.

Schucman, Helen. *A Course in Miracles.* Foundation for Inner Peace, Tiburon, Ca., 1976.

Selye, Hans. *The Stress of Life,* 2nd ed. McGraw-Hill, New York, 1978.

Shealy, C. Norman. *The Pain Game.* Celestial Arts, Berkeley, 1976.

Simonton, O. Carl, Stephanie Matthews-Simonton, and James Creighton. *Getting Well Again.* J. P. Tarcher, Los Angeles, 1978; Bantam, New York, 1980.

Schutz, Will. *Profound Simplicity.* Bantam, New York, 1979.

Solzhenitsyn, Aleksandr. *Cancer Ward,* tr. Nicholas Bethell and David Burg. Farrar, Straus & Giroux, New York, 1969; Bantam, New York, 1969.

Sveinson, Kelly. *Learning to Live with Cancer.* St. Martin's Press, New York, 1977.

Tache, J., et al. (eds.). *Cancer, Stress and Death.* Plenum Press, New York, 1979.

Totman, Richard. *Social Causes of Illness.* Pantheon, New York, 1979.

Ward, Milton. *The Brilliant Function of Pain.* Optimus Books, Plaza Hotel, New York, and CSA Press, Lakemont, Ga. 30552.

Note: Pathology numbers and reports of cases discussed are available for verification on request.

COPYRIGHT ACKNOWLEDGMENTS

About the Author

Dr. Bernard S. Siegel, who prefers to be called Bernie, not Doctor Siegel, attended Colgate University and Cornell University Medical College. He holds membership in two scholastic honor societies, Phi Beta Kappa and Alpha Omega Alpha, and graduated with honors. His surgical training took place at Yale New Haven Hospital and the Children's Hospital of Pittsburgh. He is a pediatric and general surgeon in New Haven.

In 1978 Bernie started Exceptional Cancer Patients, a specific form of individual and group therapy utilizing patients' dreams, drawings, and images. ECaP is based on "carefrontation," a loving, safe, therapeutic confrontation, which facilitates personal change and healing. This experience led to his desire to make everyone aware of his own healing potential.

The Siegel family lives in the New Haven, Connecticut, area. Bernie and his wife, Bobbie Siegel, have co-authored many articles and five children. The family has innumerable interests and pets. Their home resembles a cross between a family art gallery, zoo, museum, and automobile repair shop. In addition to conducting his very active surgical practice, Bernie now travels extensively with Bobbie to speak and run workshops sharing his techniques and experience.

Woody Allen said if he had one wish it would be to be someone else. Bernie would like to be a few inches taller.

ECaP (Exceptional Cancer Patients) is the not-for-profit, tax deductible organization founded by Dr. Siegel in 1978. In the Connecticut area, ECaP offers a clinical program with support group sessions led by psychotherapists. These are available to people who have cancer, AIDS or other life-threatening or serious chronic illnesses. In addition, each year ECaP sponsors several weekend workshops featuring Dr. Siegel that are open to anyone, with or without health problems.

ECaP has recently begun offering such services as support group facilitator training and consulting for health professionals.

ECaP has prepared packets with valuable information, including Dr. Siegel's national workshop schedule, medical information and over one hundred support service listings and ECaP-like regional referrals where they're available. This set of materials can be ordered at nominal cost ($5.00 including postage and handling).

All of the videotapes and audiocassettes featuring Dr. Siegel can be ordered through ECaP. They also carry many other unique books and tapes. To place an order, request a free catalogue of books and tapes or get additional information, please write or call:

> ECaP
> Exceptional Cancer Patients, Inc.
> 53 School Ground Road—Unit 3
> Branford, CT 06405
> phone: (203) 315-3321
> fax: (203) 315-3323

Videocassettes available featuring Dr. Siegel:

How To Be Exceptional   ECaP group members and Dr. Siegel share inspirational experiences on healing their lives. (1989)

Fight For Your Life   Informative tape with Dr. Siegel and four cancer survivors, who deliver a message of hope and determination.

Hope and a Prayer   Interview with Dr. Siegel that explores his philosophy of healing.

Innervision: Visualizing Super Health   Tape on the many uses of Visualization, featuring Dr. Siegel.

Several Lecture cassettes are available, including:

Life, Hope & Healing (1988)   A six-audiocassette set, featuring Dr. Siegel discussing in depth his philosophy and techniques for living to the fullest. Includes the stories of three survivors in their own words.

For an audio tape of *Peace, Love & Healing* or *Love, Medicine & Miracles* (abridged version) performed by Dr. Siegel on two 90-minute cassettes, contact ECaP.

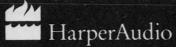

HarperAudio

A Division of HarperCollinsPublishers

LOVE, MEDICINE & MIRACLES

LOVE, MEDICINE & MIRACLES, the HarperCollins Bestseller is now available on audio-cassette read by the author, Bernie S. Siegel, M.D. In approximately three hours, Dr. Siegel guides you through his "Path of self-healing" and an exclusive meditation. PUBLISHERS WEEKLY applauded the HarperAudio offering: *"It's as if you and he are having a personal seminar."*

At your bookstore or use this convenient coupon.

Please send me the HarperAudio 2 Cassette set, LOVE, MEDICINE & MIRACLES (CPN 2107; ISBN: #0-89845-767-X). I enclose my check for $16.00 plus $3.00 per title to cover shipping and handling plus local tax where applicable.

_____ Qty. @ $16.00	$ _____
Shipping @ $3.00 per title	$ _____
Sales Tax	$ _____
Total enclosed	$ _____

For information on bulk purchases (25+ copies), please call 1-800-207-7528.

☐ If you wish to pay by check or money order, please make it payable to HarperCollins. Send your payment with this order form to HarperCollins Publishers, P.O. Box 588, Dunmore, PA 18512-0588

☐ If you wish to charge your order to a major credit card, please fill in the information below. Charge my account:

☐ American Express ☐ Visa ☐ Mastercard

Account No. _____ Expiration Date _____

Signature _____

Name _____

Address _____

City _____ State _____ Zip _____

☐ Or call 1-800-331-3761, code K00115

Please allow 4-6 weeks for delivery.